BREAKING THE CYCLE OF
opioid
addiction

BREAKING THE CYCLE OF
opioid
addiction

SUPPLEMENT YOUR PAIN MANAGEMENT
WITH CANNABIS

UWE BLESCHING

North Atlantic Books
Berkeley, CA

Published by   Cover design by Howie Severson
North Atlantic Books   Interior design by Happenstance Type-O-Rama
Berkeley, California   Printed in the United States of America

MEDICAL DISCLAIMER: The following information is intended for general information purposes only. Individuals should always see their health care provider before administering any suggestions made in this book. Any application of the material set forth in the following pages is at the reader's discretion and is his or her sole responsibility.

Breaking the Cycle of Opioid Addiction: Supplement Your Pain Management with Cannabis is sponsored and published by the Society for the Study of Native Arts and Sciences (dba North Atlantic Books), an educational nonprofit based in Berkeley, California, that collaborates with partners to develop cross-cultural perspectives, nurture holistic views of art, science, the humanities, and healing, and seed personal and global transformation by publishing work on the relationship of body, spirit, and nature.

North Atlantic Books' publications are available through most bookstores. For further information, visit our website at www.northatlanticbooks.com or call 800-733-3000.

Library of Congress Cataloging-in-Publication Data

Names: Blesching, Uwe, 1958- author.
Title: Breaking the cycle of opioid addiction : supplement your pain
    management with cannabis / Uwe Blesching ; foreword by Stephen Goldner.
Description: Berkeley, CA : North Atlantic Books, 2018. | Includes index.
Identifiers: LCCN 2017058976 (print) | LCCN 2018002770 (ebook) | ISBN
    9781623171872 (e-book) | ISBN 9781623171865 (paperback)
Subjects: LCSH: Opioid abuse—Treatment. | Cannabis—Therapeutic use. |
    Pain—Alternative treatment. | BISAC: SELF-HELP / Substance Abuse &
    Addictions / Drug Dependence. | MEDICAL / Alternative Medicine. | SOCIAL
    SCIENCE / Disease & Health Issues.
Classification: LCC RC568.O45 (ebook) | LCC RC568.O45 B54 2018 (print) | DDC
    362.29/3—dc23
LC record available at https://lccn.loc.gov/2017058976

1 2 3 4 5 6 7 8 9 SHERIDAN 23 22 21 20 19 18

Printed on recycled paper

CONTENTS

INTRODUCTION

The fabled city of San Francisco gently spreads over forty-nine rolling hills, covering seven by seven lush square miles of an exotic peninsula in Northern California. Conceived and born in the fever of the gold rush, she quickly became the prime jewel of the Pacific Coast. Her magnificent cauldron of cultures has always been a place of "high" adventure, from the whiskey saloons and opium dens of the wilder west to the cannabis-smoking Beatniks, the LSD-fueled consciousness-expanding Summer of Love, and the speedy high-tech birth of the dot-com era.

Not surprisingly, attending to an occasional drugged patient was part and parcel of my work as a paramedic for the San Francisco Department of Public Health. However, from the early 1990s on, I began to notice a not-so-subtle change among patients needing emergency assistance.[1]

It became increasingly rare for a shift to pass without getting a dispatch about someone unconscious and not breathing. One patient prone on the sidewalk in the Tenderloin, another crouched over in a public restroom on Mission Street, or yet another falling off a bench in Golden Gate Park. However, there were peak times when a new batch of drugs had entered the streets of San Francisco. No one knew the exact composition, concentration, or quantity to take to get the desired effects. It was in those days that overdoses (ODs) were really common.

There were the usual telltale signs. Pinpoint pupils, pale skin, bluish lips or nail beds, a shallow but rapid pulse. An absent or agonizing respiratory effort on the part of the patient. Needle paraphernalia. Fresh or old needle marks. A wet crotch from melting ice cubes placed there by a concerned friend. I always wondered if that ever worked, or was it just an urban myth? And while I never discovered the truth about ice cubes in the pants, I did learn a lot about opioids—the good, the bad, and the ugly. I learned a lot about what addiction looks like. I learned a lot about pain. I learned what worked and what didn't on the job. One of the early lessons was patience and attention to details.

The problem, from a paramedic's perspective, is that opioids *(o-pee-oyds)* such as morphine, oxycodone, and heroin bind to opioid receptors in the brain and, depending on the dose or concentration, can cause sedation so intense that the body simply stops any effort to breathe. The opioid antidote is called Narcan, a brand name for naloxone. When it is injected and enters the bloodstream, it quickly reaches the opioid receptors, knocks the heroin or other opioid loose, and immediately takes its place, thus reversing all physical ill effects.

This remarkable transformation occurred very quickly if I was lucky enough to find a workable vein, a bit slower if I had to inject into a muscle. Eventually, either within seconds or within minutes, the patient gasped for air, opened his eyes, and returned from his near-death experience. However, if I was impatient and not attuned to the slow and subtle responses and injected more Narcan to force a more rapid therapeutic result, I ended up injecting enough of the antidote to induce instant withdrawal symptoms in the patient. With the patient now suddenly awake, I was faced with an angry, irritable, aching person who usually and somewhat correctly held me responsible for his ill-fated misfortunes. Inevitably, the fact did not register that mere seconds earlier he was unconscious and in respiratory arrest, minutes or seconds away from death or brain death. Thus I learned the hard way not to be too hasty or too generous with Narcan. I also learned that when the temporary curtain of opioid-based pain relief is pulled back quickly and completely, a raw, tangled web of pain takes its place front and center stage.

It turned out that being slow and deliberate made me keenly aware of my patient's individual circumstances. On the surface was the struggle, the compulsion, the lack of control, the aggression, the lawlessness, and irritability. Yet just beneath the surface was a thinly concealed deeper reality of omnipresent pain (physical, mental, and emotional) expressed in loss of meaningful connection and resulting loneliness, in shame and feelings of worthlessness, or in the shadow of utter despair or hopelessness.

One day a young lawyer whom we will call Gene had overdosed at home, and when he awoke after the Narcan ritual he was miserable and in pain. He wanted to use the bathroom to relieve himself before we left for the ER. When he opened the door and came back out I smelled the unmistakable scent of freshly burned cannabis. Gene suggested that he was fine and didn't need to go to the hospital. I checked him out, and indeed, he looked fine. His vital signs were stable, he was lucid, and his physical pain and irritability had diminished. He articulated (and I am paraphrasing) that he was just doing heroin to feel OK enough to function, that he had been doing it for seven years to keep the mostly mental and emotional pain at bay, and that he wasn't addicted.

At first I didn't think too much about it. After all, when you work in the emergency medical services (EMS), pain is all around you. For twenty-four hours straight, seven days a week, with no breaks on holidays, pain is everywhere. From one call to the next, you are thrust into another person's worst time of their life. Sadly, even outside the extremes of EMS, too often pain is omnipresent in some way. And it seems to be getting worse today.

The use of prescription opioid analgesia alone has doubled over a period of ten years (2000–2010),[2] with nearly a third of the entire U.S. population now using opioids. Think about it. And this is only one number; it does not include other pain medication or the use of opioids obtained in ways other than a legal physician-issued prescription.

What is truly horrific is that the consumption of a mountain of painkillers does not appear to improve patient conditions, health, and well-being in the long run.[3] The scope of lingering pain, the ongoing damage inflicted on body, mind, and emotions, the growing number of accidental deaths, and the associated societal costs are truly staggering. Such a high mountain also casts a very long shadow. Nearly everyone using opioids experiences some form of adverse effects. Some of them are on the milder side, such as constipation or itching, while others are more harmful in their nature, such as the suppression of one's breath, with a potentially fatal outcome, and the high potential for addiction in certain individuals.

Here, too, the facts speak for themselves. Drug overdose deaths in the United States exceeded 64,000 in 2016, the majority of them (53,332) being opioid-related deaths.[4] Nearly 80 percent of heroin users started with prescription opioids.[5] The gateway drugs to heroin are pharmaceutical opioids.[6] But are opioids solely responsible for all this misery? The current evidence accumulated so far is insufficient and even contradictory in chronicling the actual risk of prescription opioid-based addiction rates, with estimates ranging between less than 1 percent to 56 percent.[7]

In direct contrast to the shadow side of opioid use are those patients who use opioids even for long periods of time and do not become addicted.[8] So the emerging question is, why do some people get addicted while others don't? What makes a person vulnerable to becoming addicted? What fortifies another, and what makes someone seemingly immune to addiction?

The opioid-related addiction and death crisis and the complex and underlying questions are not answered nor effectively addressed by the traditional and orthodox approaches. In fact, orthodox medicine is struggling to understand and correct how patients in need of effective pain control end up addicted and dying from those pills meant to help in the first place.

Over time I thought a lot about Gene the lawyer. It occurred to me that Gene might have demonstrated a novel solution to therapeutically address the pain of acute opioid withdrawal symptoms. It wasn't until years later when I was doing research for my PhD—and my first book on the topic, *The Cannabis Health Index*—that a scientific foundation for the development of cannabis or cannabinoid-based products to therapeutically mitigate the opioid abuse crisis began to appear on the horizon.

In fact, solutions are already available, and as you will see, they are not going to be black or white, pro or con, for or against, but instead require a more nuanced and holistic approach to dealing with the complex web of pain residing behind the curtain of opioid use and opioid addiction.

For instance, feelings such as pain (in body, mind, or emotions) drive addiction and recovery, and it can be argued that one of the most promising approaches to date started twenty-five years ago when Raphael Mechoulam and his team of international researchers poured the foundation for the modern cannabinoid health sciences. He mused: "We believed then—and still do—that the endocannabinoid system plays a role in the formation of emotions."[9]

Fast forward to now. States that allow for medicinal cannabis saw a 25 percent drop in opioid deaths,[10] and more and more patients are switching from opioid-based analgesia to cannabis for effective and safe pain management and resolution.[11] Or consider Portugal, the innovative European country that has created a completely new paradigm for addressing drug abuse and the underlying and driving physical, mental, and emotional pain—it is a supportive approach that is in direct opposition to the War on Drugs. As a result, the nation's total overdose death rate dropped by 80 percent since changes were implemented in 2001, saving and improving untold individual lives and enhancing overall societal quality of life.[12]

Informed by the latest discoveries and insights from pain and addiction research as well as the cannabinoid health sciences, this book makes a case for utilizing cannabis to supplement pain management and to help mitigate opioid withdrawal symptoms. By understanding the strengths and limitations of opioids and cannabinoids and the science behind the pain-addiction connection, the reader will be able to identify individual root causes and develop practical steps to prevent or break the cycle of opioid addiction.

one

The Opioid Crisis: Where We Are and How We Got Here

Mistakes are, after all, the foundations of truth, and if a man does not know what a thing is, it is at least an increase in knowledge if he knows what it is not.

—CARL JUNG

ABOUT A THIRD OF the U.S. population suffers from chronic debilitating pain.[13] Thus it should come as no surprise that opioids are the most commonly prescribed analgesics (painkillers) in the country. In 2012, U.S. pharmacies alone filled 289 million opioid prescriptions for the current population of 320 million.[14] In fact, the U.S. consumes more than 50 percent of the global supply of morphine.[15] This indisputable reality is especially puzzling when we consider the scientific evidence showing that long-term opioid therapy for chronic pain has a very limited efficacy.[16] The takeaway? We are a country with a lot of people in pain. It is a stubborn kind of pain that resists and persists. Opioids alone do not provide the complete or lasting healing that clearly so many patients need and are looking for. And these powerful drugs come with side effects and a risk of addiction and overdose death.

Today it is estimated that more than ten million people using prescription opioids have begun to use them for purposes other than prescribed,[17] such as blunting mental-emotional anguish or the pains that come with opioid withdrawal symptoms. As such, a significant number of them are feared addicted. While exact statistics are difficult to obtain, the American Society for Addiction Medicine estimates that about two million people have an opioid substance-use disorder.[18] For far too many, prescription opioids have become the gateway to the use of heroin (the street version of opioids),[19] and estimates of people with heroin addiction in the United States approach 600,000.[20] Perhaps the discrepancy between 10 million "nonmedical" users and the combined 2.6 million people considered to have a substance-use disorder using either prescription opioids or heroin can be explained in part by the fact that not everybody who uses opioids gets addicted.[21] So if the drugs are not the sole determining factor in addiction, what are the personal vulnerabilities that lead to and underlie it? It's a question mostly ignored by U.S. policies.

Current governmental efforts to counter addiction are lukewarm and weakly funded, if they are funded at all. While they seldom meaningfully address the roots of the problem of drug abuse and addiction, these efforts are somewhat helpful. They include prevention, treatment, and harm reduction (needle exchanges, safe injection sites, opioid substitution therapies). In contrast, law enforcement and global assistance for eradication (think poppy fields in Asia) receive the bulk of political and taxpayer-funded support. Unfortunately, the moneyed solutions we have been throwing at addiction generate little success in overcoming the epidemic. The lack of well-thought-out and effective approaches contributes to the unenlightened state of affairs we find ourselves in today. Much of the public debate about drug addiction is based on decades-old information and long-held yet baseless attitudes, resulting in black-and-white judgments that reveal thinly disguised prejudices[22] and unexamined biases.[23] It's a short hop from there to unhelpful finger-pointing, along with rigid adherence to incomplete or discredited models of addiction. Such models offer little if any innovation and primarily serve to maintain the failed and expensive prohibition policies of the long-standing War on Drugs.

Pharmaceutical opioids, including heroin,[24] have become more potent, greatly increasing all risks associated with inappropriate use. For example, one of the most potent versions is carfentanil, a fentanyl analog, which can be 10,000 times more powerful than morphine.[25] Think of it this way: the tiniest amount, a microgram (a grain the size of salt), is enough to induce adverse effects in humans, making it very difficult for illicit products to be measured in small enough doses to prevent near-instant respiratory arrest. While carfentanil (trade name Wildnil) is supposed to be used as an anesthetic for large animals such as elephants, it is readily available for purchase on the internet. Acting Director of the U.S. Drug Enforcement Agency Chuck Rosenberg issued a recent warning to public service agencies and the public: "Carfentanil is surfacing in more and more communities."[26] Resulting death from all types of opioid overdose has reached epidemic proportions, with more than one hundred people needlessly dying every day.[27] The opioid crisis does not discriminate, and no part of society has proven immune: soccer moms, farmers, the homeless and the 1 percent, radio talk-show hosts, lawyers, carpenters, and physicians. And this trend is rapidly growing.

This is where we are today. The good news is that it doesn't have to be this way. But before we look at emerging solutions to more effective relief of pain in all its dimensions and the opioid crisis in all its manifestations, it is helpful to examine when and how the current crisis began.

A Most Influential Letter

How did we get here? What happened that well-meaning physicians, dedicated to alleviating pain and suffering, began prescribing opioids that literally started killing a large number of their patients all across the great divide? What happened that patients who were seeking an end to their pain and suffering found themselves caught in a chronic loop of pain? And how did a number of them with vulnerabilities to developing addictions get hooked on pills they thought would heal their pain?

It may seem silly, but it can be argued that it all started with a letter that was inked in 1980. Until that time, most opioid use was informed by the decades-long practice initiated by the Harrison Narcotics Act of 1914.[28] Physicians as well as many patients were well aware of and concerned about the risks of opiate use.* The drugs were primarily used in acute cases—injury,

---

* While the terms are becoming interchangeable today, *opiates* referred to plant-derived medicines in this family; the term *opioids* was adopted later to distinguish artificial versions of the poppy plant's natural medicine.

surgery, and significant end-of-life illness and suffering—and only for relatively short periods of time. The letter published in the widely read *New England Journal of Medicine* was written by Jane Porter and Hershel Jick, and it was titled "Addiction Rare in Patients Treated with Narcotics."

Thirty-seven years later, a team of Canadian researchers performed a bibliometric analysis on that very letter and discovered that this "five-sentence letter published in the *Journal* in 1980 was heavily and uncritically cited as evidence that addiction was rare with long-term opioid therapy. We believe that this citation pattern contributed to the North American opioid crisis by helping to shape a narrative that allayed prescribers' concerns about the risk of addiction associated with long-term opioid therapy."[29]

The letter may have been initially well intended to serve a growing population with chronic pain, but it quickly produced a paradigm shift in opioid prescription protocols that contributed to the current opioid crisis. The study identified a total of 608 citations since the letter's publication, with a significant increase in letter citation on par with the introduction of OxyContin to the U.S. market. A majority of authors cited the letter as evidence that addiction was rare in patients treated with opioids, while others grossly misrepresented the conclusions of the letter, and this helped to build undeserved confidence.[30] A number of influential organizations and allied professors were able to shift physician opinion and treatment protocols in practice. During this time, an aggressive marketing campaign was launched by Purdue Pharma, promising that its product, OxyContin, could give pain relief with lower risk of abuse or addiction than other opioids.

On May 10, 2007, Purdue Pharma and three of its executives pleaded guilty in federal court on charges related to misleading physicians, regulators, and patients about the addiction risk potential of their opioid OxyContin. The company agreed to pay $600 million in fines to federal and state agencies and to settle litigation brought by patients harmed by the inaccurate claims.[31] Since then, other opioid makers, including Johnson & Johnson, McKesson, and Teva, and their distributors, including Walgreens, Walmart, and CVS, have faced an increasing number of lawsuits brought by a growing number of U.S. cities and counties in California, New York, and Illinois as well as First Nations such as the Cherokee Nation and state governments such as Ohio,

Oklahoma, and Tennessee for damages done to human lives and the collective wallet. Allow me to give you just one example of the latter.

Narcan (naloxone) is the prime antidote for an opioid overdose. In my past work as a paramedic, I used it a thousand and one times to wake up patients so deeply sedated that their bodies had stopped breathing. A low-concentration opioid such as heroin, for example, may require 1 or 2 mg of intravenous Narcan to quickly reverse the harmful effects. On the other hand, fentanyl or its analogs may require so much Narcan that we would need to dispatch another unit because we ran out of supplies. Unchecked free markets allowed producers to raise the cost of this simple life-saving compound up to 500 percent, cashing in while local governments were left facing ever-increasing need and cost.[32] Increasing Narcan availability to the public and reducing its cost are commonly recognized as significant components of harm-reduction strategies.[33]

The Plot Thickens— Other Contributing Factors

In addition to the often quoted and unsubstantiated letter in an influential journal, the opioid crisis was fueled by a number of other factors, such as incentives for prescribing doctors in the form of money, gifts, or travel, for example. While this practice was banned by the Physician Payments Sunshine Act of 2009,[34] it was in full operational swing in the preceding years, further shifting practice toward a more abundant use of opioids.

With the allure of exotic trips and gifts now under scrutiny, opioid makers devised a different strategy to further tilt opinion about and use of opioids. For instance, the U.S. General Accounting Office reported in 2003:

> In addition to expanding its sales force, Purdue used multiple approaches to market and promote OxyContin. These approaches included expanding its physician speaker bureau and conducting speaker training conferences, sponsoring pain-related educational programs, issuing OxyContin starter coupons for patients' initial prescriptions, sponsoring pain-related websites, advertising OxyContin in medical journals, and distributing OxyContin marketing items to health care professionals.

Another element contributing to the conditions for the perfect storm of our opioid crisis is the decrease in multidisciplinary pain clinics that in 1980 were actually popular and measurably successful.[35] The growth of managed care and a move toward the use of an accounting model called current procedural terminology codes (CPT for short), designed to charge per service, led to the separation of a complex and combined approach to dealing with chronic pain that had worked well for many in the past. Instead, pharmaceutical (opioid and nonopioid) and procedure-based subspecialties for chronic pain (such as nerve blocks, epidural cortisol injections, and spinal fusion) emerged that fit nicely with the fee-for-service model. Studies comparing the results of this shift in handling chronic pain have determined that patients got worse and costs increased.[36]

In 1996, about the same time that OxyContin was approved for marketing by the Federal Drug Administration (FDA), a well-meaning new concept, "pain as the fifth vital sign," was introduced by the American Pain Society.[37] It was at first adopted by the Veterans Health Administration and the Joint Commission on accreditation of health care organizations. From their highly respected platforms, it was widely accepted and used across the nation. The new national trend involved addressing a patient's pain on par with changes in other vital signs (blood pressure, heart rate, respiratory rate, and body temperature). It carried a noticeable, well-documented, and unintended consequence—a rise in use of prescription opioids and a rise in opioid-related addiction and death.

You might wonder why the FDA, charged with protecting patients from misleading marketing claims, failed to prevent the crisis. Scott Gottlieb, the FDA administrator appointed much later, said at his confirmation hearings in April 2017 that the FDA had been "complicit, even if unwittingly," in creating the opioid epidemic. The FDA, he suggested, "didn't fully recognize the scope of the emerging problem," and he wanted to develop a new approach.[38] What specifically Gottlieb was referring to is unclear, but it might have to do with cases such as OxyContin or Opana, for example.

After all, the FDA approved OxyContin for marketing. Did they not figure out that the manufacturers made misleading claims now proven in court? In a related case, the opioid Opana was first approved by the FDA for marketing in 2006. However, as abuse reports came in, the manufacturing company Endo in 2010 resubmitted a new formulation of Opana that was designed to be resistant to the physical or chemical manipulation used to turn the oral drug into one that could be injected or snorted (making it more easily a drug of abuse). Reformulated Opana was approved in 2011, but the FDA did not allow Endo to market the drug as one resistant to abuse. In 2015 Opana was held responsible for an outbreak of HIV, hepatitis C, and a serious blood disorder (thrombotic microangiopathy) in rural Indiana after people shared needles with contents made from Opana.[39] In 2017, at the request of the FDA, Endo withdrew Opana from the market.[40]

Another contributing factor that got us to where we are today is the emergence of "pill mills." These are pain clinics, doctor's offices, or health care facilities that prescribe opioids for basically any reason. You get to choose what opioids you prefer. Patients are often in and out without a physical examination but with a prescription or with actual opioids in their hands or directions to complicit pharmacies. Transactions are done mostly in cash. Pill mills tend to render opioid analgesic services and usually few if any other procedures. They often move from place to place in rapid succession to avoid prosecution. In 2008 the top five opioid-prescribing locations were Nevada, Delaware, Florida, Kentucky, and Tennessee.[41] The DEA has made some progress is closing pill mills. For instance, in 2013 the DEA Public Information Officer announced:

> In 2010, the Drug Enforcement Administration's (DEA) Automation of Reports and Consolidated Orders System (ARCOS) reported that 90 of the top 100 oxycodone-purchasing physicians in the nation were located in Florida. The number of Florida doctors appearing in that nationwide list dropped from 90 to only 13 in 2011. Today the DEA is happy to announce that there are no Florida doctors on this list.[42]

When pill mills leave, patients turn to what is left—street heroin or cyber pharmacies. Generally referred to as vendors of the Dark Web, cyber-pharmacies such as AlphaBay or Silk Road marketplace build an intricate operation to supply opioids to consumers around the globe. They commonly use cryptocurrencies such as Bitcoin to avoid detection, and they might employ suppliers from one country, carry out banking in another, and deliver to yet another. When the U.S. Department of Justice announced the results of an international sting together with police agencies from Canada, Thailand, Holland, Britain, Lithuania, and France, they had found over 200,000 users and more than 40,000 purveyors of opioids and other illicit goods.[43]

As you can see, while it may have started with a simple published letter, there were numerous factors that contributed to creating the current opioid crisis. And any novel approach will need to be multilayered and complex to mitigate and eventually end the crisis. The good thing is we don't have to wait for the world to change. A number of practical and effective things can be done now to make a real difference in our lives and in the lives of those we love and care for. To lay the foundation for a new approach to addressing pain, opioids, and addiction, it helps to look at the history of opioid use in all its form and manifestations—the good, the bad, and the ugly.

two

The History and Science of Opioids, in Brief

Everything one does in life, even love, occurs in an express train racing toward death. To smoke opium is to get out of the train while it is still moving. It is to concern oneself with something other than death.

—JEAN COCTEAU

OPIUM-BASED DRUGS ARE THE single class of compounds gifted by nature with the ability to relieve more suffering than any other medication in the known history of humankind. Physicians of old were well aware of opium's capacity to take away pain and were careful to avoid potential adverse effects due to inappropriate use.[44] It is noteworthy that records from ancient history show the abundant, liberal, and routine usage of opium but no evidence of the widespread problems with addiction[45] that are so prevalent in more recent histories, from roughly the late eighteenth century to the present. In other words, opiates have been used for thousands of years and abused for about two centuries. Opioids—the modern term— are opium-emulating compounds, many of which have been formulated relatively recently. Sometimes you will see the spelling *opiates,* which was used to differentiate a plant-based version from an artificial (opioid) form. However, for the purpose of this book, the terms are synonymous and used interchangeably.

I for one do not fault opium, for I have come to believe that the miracle of opium—its superpower, if you will—lies in its ability to grant reprieve from the intensity of pain. Its power, however, does not extend to resolving pain; it can only buy us a little time for our bodies to heal and for our psyche to integrate the pain and the underlying trauma. In this way we are ideally able to learn from the experience, give it meaning, or to provide context that allows for the transcendence of pain. The compassionate function of opium is perhaps a reminder that life doesn't have to be this painful.

The Opium Poppy: True Flower Power

Due to extensive global cultivation practices dating back to the earliest memories of human history, no one knows for sure where the opium poppy originated. Today the plant is native on every continent with the exception of Antarctica.[46]

The poppy family (Papaveraceae) contains more than forty genera and hundreds of species (these are taxonomic ranks). One of them is *Papaver somniferum*, the opium poppy. *Papaver* is derived from the Latin word for "poppy," and *somniferum* is a combination of the Latin *somnus* for "sleep" and *fer*, meaning "to carry." There are numerous subspecies with a variety of visual appearances and plant constituents, and each may contain different quantities of analgesic compounds. However, *Papaver somniferum* is the single poppy species that contains the most abundant amounts. A white latex-like juice exudes whenever the plant is wounded. The latex is especially concentrated in the seedpods and contains numerous biologically active alkaloids such as codeine and, of course, morphine. The latex is the opium.

Some of the distinctive properties that allow you to discern that you are working with *Papaver somniferum* are: The plant can be taller than three feet. Flowers usually consist of four petals presenting in red, white, mauve, or light purple. The color themes sometimes thicken toward the petal base to reveal a darker shade of one of its base colors. The stem and leaves are bluish-gray-green in appearance and are covered in short wiry hair. The emerging central seedpod at the center of the flower is surrounded by an abundant swarm of stamens (the fertilizing organ of a flower) covered in grayish pollen. Once the seed pods are fully formed, they tend to be on the larger side (one inch or more). They are smooth, spherical capsules surrounded by vertical rays forming a crown-like flat top with small openings. The seeds themselves often take on a bluish-black color.

In week two after blooming, after the petals have fallen off, the harvest starts. Opium farmers begin the repetitive, exhausting, back-breaking task, unchanged for millennia, of making shallow vertical cuts, pin pricks, or v-shaped incisions in the outer layer of skin of the unripe seed pods. This occurs over a period of several days. The white latex soon oozes out, forming sticky droplets as it dries over a few hours and turns brown due to exposure to the air. A dull blade is used to scrape the brown sticky opium, which is then collected pod by pod by hand and worked into lumps that do not rot and are virtually imperishable.

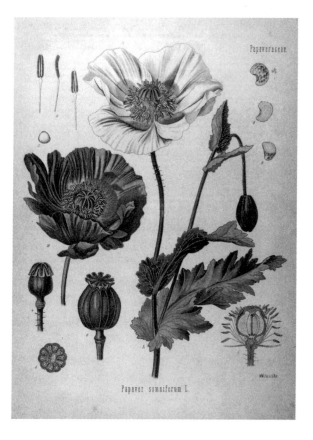

Evidence of Opium Use from the Ancient World

While most people associate opium with the Far East, there is no mention in ancient Sanskrit, Brahmanical, Buddhist, or Jinist literature.[47] Further, as you will see, archeological evidence suggests that its more recent historical use and popularity likely originated and spread from the classical Mediterranean cultures to Europe, Egypt, Arabia, Southeast Asia, East Asia, and the rest of the world.

The most ancient mention of the poppy is given on a small white clay tablet excavated near Nippur, south of modern-day Baghdad, the spiritual center of the Sumerians.[48] Author C. E. Terry states in his 1928 book that he "was informed by Professor R. Dougherty, Curator of the Babylonian Collection at Yale University, that opium must have been known to the Sumerians because they had an ideogram, 'Hul Gil,' corresponding to this drug."[49] This apparently was known to Harry G. Anslinger, the first Commissioner of the Federal Bureau of Narcotics, and William F. Tompkins, U.S. Attorney for the District of New Jersey, who wrote on page 1 of their 1953 book *The Traffic in Narcotics*:

> On the clay tablets of the Sumerians it was recorded that the juice of the poppy was "collected in the early morning," perhaps before the Eastern sun should have tempered its anodyne (analgesic). This people of the land of Sumer in lower Mesopotamia—now the Arab kingdom of Iraq—cultivated the poppy plant five thousand years BC in order to extract its juice; *gil* was the name they gave it, which translated means joy or rejoicing, and this name is still used today for opium in some parts of the world.[50]

It is likely that the Assyrians and Babylonians, successors of the Sumerian civilization, learned how to culture opium and use it for medicinal and spiritual purposes. It appears to have spread from there west toward Egypt and east toward Persia.

Physical evidence includes artifacts from archeological excavations that suggest widespread opium use for healing and spiritual purposes as early as the fifteenth century BCE in the eastern Mediterranean and Crete.[51] A particularly beautiful sculpture of the Minoan *Goddess of Poppies* (her crown is made from poppy pods) from that era survived the assault of the ages and is visible in all her splendor in the Archeological Museum in Heraklion, Crete. In reverence to the analgesic and anesthetic properties of opium, she has become the symbol of the Department of Anesthesiology of the University of Crete.[52]

Based on the discovery of an ointment containing morphine found in the tomb of the eighteenth-dynasty Egyptian pharaohs (1550–1292 BCE), which included the reign of Tutankhamen, archeologists date the use of poppies or opium-based products to at least that time. According to texts found, the flowers were called *shepenndšr* and the seed pods *sheppen*.[53]

A historical blink of an eye later, the poppy shows up in the writings of the Greek poet Hesiod in the eighth century BCE, who mentions a city named Mekonê, or "Poppy Town."[54] The poppy is described growing in the gardens of Hekatê near Kolchis in the fabled story of Jason and the Argonauts,[55] and it is mentioned by Homer in both the *Iliad* and *Odyssey*.[56] It has been claimed that Alexander the Great on his epic march with his army and attending physicians first introduced opium to Southeast Asia, but confirming records are wanting, while the time of the Roman empire was ripe with records of the therapeutic properties of opium.[57]

Researchers of plants mentioned in the Bible and Talmud suggest that the reference in the scriptures to "gall" indicates poppy juice. It was called *rosh* in Hebrew and was added to the vinegar that the Hebrews gave to Christ on the cross in order to relieve his suffering.[58] One direct reference to opium in the Talmud can be found under the name *ophion*.[59] About the time of Christ, Egyptian opium was produced and traded in Thebes and called Theban opium, which would get a twentieth-century nod in the name of the opioid thebaine.

Opium in the West: Mystery and Medicine

The word *opium* is derived from the Greek word *opos,* simply meaning the sap of the poppy pods.[60] Far from the innocent, descriptive, and original meaning, the term *opium* quickly evolved to take on more complex, shadowy, and contradictory evocations. Some were reflective of its mental-emotional properties, such as euphoria, ecstasy, or voluptuous arousal, while others were more indicative of the physical impact, such as sleep, sedation, or death.

The therapeutic application of opium in the Christian era first shows up historically in written records associated with Hippocrates,[61] the father of modern medicine (see the Hippocratic oath), who mentions its hypnotic, narcotic, and cathartic properties, as did Aristotle.[62] The Aesculapian physician Galen (second century CE) wrote: "Opium is the strongest of the drugs that numb the senses and induce a deadening sleep."[63]

After the fall of the Roman Empire (fifth century CE), opium use largely disappeared from Europe. During the medieval period or Dark Ages—the fifth through fifteenth centuries CE, an era that saw the Crusades and the Inquisition—public perception from the patriarchy down viewed anything associated with the East as suspect of affiliation with demons or the devil. The medicinal use of opium was strictly frowned upon, as pain was seen as God-given, and therefore interference would be considered blasphemous and suspected of witchcraft. This is not to say that opium wasn't secretly used in some circles with access to traders from the East.

It wasn't until the sixteenth century that Swiss physician and alchemist Paracelsus explored opium's properties. He is generally credited with reintroducing opium to Europe in some notable capacity. Full-spectrum opium alkaloids (whole-plant opium) were dissolved in alcohol and named laudanum, after the Latin word *laudare,* meaning "to praise." These liquids were once again acknowledged and used as medicine in Europe. Laudanum became very popular in the following century when the English physician Thomas Sydenham (1624–1689) popularized his version of it, Laudanum de Sydenham, a tincture of opium mixed with the spices cinnamon, saffron, and clove.[64]

Laudanum and other opioid-based preparations have been (and in some cases still are) a remedy for a variety of indications, such as pain and painful conditions (rheumatoid arthritis, gout, menstrual difficulties, teething, and piles, a.k.a. hemorrhoids), cough (pleurisy; tuberculosis, a.k.a. consumption; and whooping cough), diarrhea, insomnia, heart disease, and spasms and other alcohol-withdrawal symptoms (such as seizures and delirium tremens). It was especially popular to prescribe laudanum for perceived "female troubles" such as "hysteria," "fainting fits," "mood swings," anxiety, or depression, for example. Famous Victorian writers who used laudanum include Charles Dickens, author of numerous classics such as *The Adventures of Oliver Twist;* Bram Stoker, the author of *Dracula;* and poet and activist Elizabeth Barrett Browning, who published *The Cry of the Children,* attacking child labor practices of that time.

Opium was a household staple in the early American colonies, after the *Mayflower* arrived in 1620. It was openly cultivated in the New World, its resin mixed with whiskey and cherished as an effective treatment for coughs and pains.[65] Thomas Jefferson (1742–1826), who suffered greatly from chronic diarrhea, used laudanum, which enabled him to return to the out-of-doors and his love of horseback riding.[66] He cultivated *Papaver somniferum* on his estate.[67]

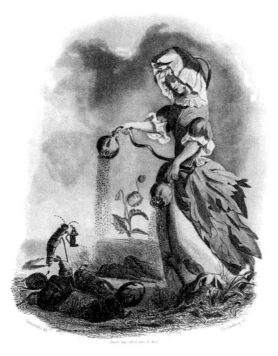

The author of one of the first books written on the subject of opium, in 1793, considered addiction as a possibility, including a mention of withdrawal symptoms, but this did not lead him to issue a warning for either its recreational or medicinal use.[68] And while there are historical reports signaling the possibility of habituations to opium by this point in time (roughly the end of the eighteenth century), there are no accounts of widespread addiction associated with the use of opium as medicine.[69] However, things were already changing in both the Far East and the West, with addiction on the rise.

In 1816, a milestone event occurred in science-based medicine when the German pharmacist Friedrich W. A. Sertürner isolated an individual compound—one of the key analgesic alkaloids—from the totality of the opium poppy's constituents. Sertürner promptly and aptly named it *morphine* after the Greek god of dreams, Morpheus. He recorded his process (pharmacological properties, crystallization, crystalline structure, and analyses) in a scientific paper that changed the world of medicine.[70] His process ushered in not just the modern usage of one of the most important medicines of our time but also a new era of isolating lifesaving and life-sustaining medicinal compounds that became the basis for modern pharmacological medicine.

By the mid to late 1820s, morphine was becoming famous for its analgesic properties and was readily available in hospitals in the United States and Europe. The Civil War (1861–1865) saw the first large-scale application of oral opium and injectable morphine, bringing relief to thousands of battle-injured soldiers and civilians alike.

Over time, more alkaloids were found and isolated from opium. For instance, codeine (methyl-morphine), named after the Greek word *kodeia,* meaning "poppy head," was isolated by the French chemist Pierre-Jean Robiquet in 1832.[71] Heroin (diamorphine), ultimately named after the German word *heroisch* (synonym of *heldenhaft*), meaning "strong," "bold," and "heroic" in reference to its ability to allay pain, was initially isolated from morphine in 1874 by the British chemist Charles Romley Alder Wright[72] and later in 1887 rediscovered or resynthesized by the German chemist Felix Hoffmann, working for Farbenfabriken, later Bayer.[73] Bayer brought heroin to the market in 1898 as an over-the-counter medication, presented as a nonaddictive alternative to morphine,[74] a painkiller, sedative, and antitussive (cough medicine).

The late nineteenth century gave birth to the heroin paradox. Among the standard indications, heroin was initially considered safer than morphine.[75] Indeed, it was thought to be helpful in alleviating symptoms of morphine withdrawal.[76] It wasn't until a decade or so later that it was generally realized that heroin also caused addiction-related problems in certain individuals. With the passing of the Harrison Narcotics Tax Act in 1914, the government started to channel and control heroin and other opioids more tightly, through physician prescriptions only. By 1924 heroin was banned, and today heroin (like cannabis) is a Schedule I substance, officially deemed to have no medical value.

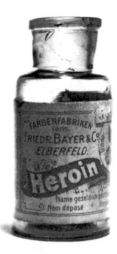

It is perhaps noteworthy that until the 1850s, opioids were primarily administered orally, limiting their therapeutic potential to those patients who could swallow and keep them down, as well as limiting their efficacy via alterations by digestive juices in the stomach and when passing the liver and bile ducts. In 1853 the first effective, precise, and reliable syringe was developed by the Scottish physician Alexander Wood,[77] after which injecting opioids quickly became the norm.

Opium Wars in the Far East

Traditionally, opium was an herbal remedy that was ingested, not smoked. For example, its use during China's Ming dynasty (1368–1644) was legal and focused primarily on medicinal applications such as the treatment of pain. Opium's use later (mid-Ming) transformed and expanded to a popular aphrodisiac and luxury item for the Ming emperor, his favorite consorts, government officials, and scholarly elites.[78] This was when smoking the substance became a more widespread practice.

With the emergence of the Qing dynasty (a.k.a. Ch'ing or Manchu dynasty, 1644–1912), China slowly ushered in the longest-lasting and richest period in dynastic history. During the Qing dynasty, the nation's population grew by three hundred million in a relatively short period of time, and China was able to sustain this population in widespread prosperity. The Middle Kingdom advanced traditional approaches to life, producing tremendous growth in many arenas, including agriculture, philosophy, and the arts, which included porcelain, silk, and literature. It was in this period of prosperity that it became popular and practical for the middle and working classes to emulate the elite and to smoke opium as a social and recreational practice.

The Dutch and Portuguese established early trade networks offering opium grown in India to feed the emerging demand for it in China. Fueled by the loose purse strings (actually silver coins) of considerable numbers of people with disposable income, the opium enterprise turned extremely profitable. A popular way to smoke opium was to mix it with tobacco and other herbs in a concoction called *madak*. However, when commoners took to opium, the perception of the elites began to shift. Opium slowly came to be viewed in the Middle Kingdom as vulgar or common.

The British Empire took notice of this profitable activity and wanted not just a piece of the opium pie—it wanted it all. It forced the Bengali opium

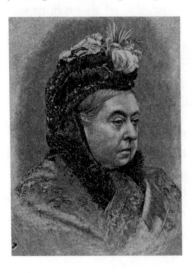

growers into servitude, and through the British East India Company, the English bullied their way into the opium market with military force and took control. Thus Britain, and Queen Victoria, would become the most prolific drug dealers in the world.

By 1729, smoking *madak* was becoming politicized and associated with so-called rebels concentrating along the southern coast of China. It was a serious enough potential problem that the Emperor Yongzheng made it illegal to smoke or sell *madak*.[79] The ban was ineffectual. Chinese efforts to enforce the ban on opium led the British to declare war. In the first Opium War (1839–1842), Britain technologically out-maneuvered the Chinese, with Navy gunboats inflicting heavy casualties for the Qing and eventually forcing the Chinese to give up on prohibition. In this settlement, Hong Kong became part of the British Empire. In the second Opium War (1856–1860), the British were joined by the French. It culminated in the final Battle of Tongzhou, in which the Qing soldiers took heavy losses. And it was here, at this point in time, as a consequence of forced imposition of free trade of opium, that widespread addiction truly took hold and began to produce the immense social pain and problems that were part and parcel of the final years of decline of the Qing dynasty. This period is considered by many Chinese as "the century of shame," which didn't end until the Chinese communists came to power in 1949.

The Modern Culture of Hopelessness

In contrast to China, a different kind of socioeconomic and political upheaval was triggered by the Industrial Revolution (1750–1850) on the other side of the world, which brought often-painful changes to large sections of the British population. People lost their old way of life as they went from working in the fields or around the home to laboring in factories, mines, textile mills, or offices upon relocating to cities. Workdays lasted up to sixteen hours. Child labor was rampant, the physical toll extreme, and wages low. For better or worse, men lost their patriarchal role and identity as the head of the household, as all family members, including women and children, were now serving the owners of factories or mills. Mothers were forced to leave infants alone at home and turned to laudanum or laudanum-like preparations to pacify their little offspring, leading to infant mortality rates as high as 16 percent.[80] How is a person to cope with such chronically painful, drastic, and sudden changes to body, mind, and emotions? As in the case of China, it is easy to posit that self-medicating with opium was an attempt to cope in the face of overwhelming stressors such as hopelessness, alienation, and the sense of powerlessness.

For far too many, the conditions of the past that contributed to vulner-abilities to addiction are still in place today—such as severe and confusing social changes, growing unemployment, poverty, income inequity, loss of meaning and dignity, and hopelessness, along with its ever-present physical and mental pain.

You may want to take note of one of the first studies to examine poten-tial causes for the recent increase in drug-related deaths; it was conducted by the National Health Services of Scotland in 2017. Its results and conclu-sions mirror the portraits of many rural and suburban areas in the United States. The analysis shows that the increase in addiction-related deaths may be explained by rampant erosion of hope in certain depressed communities, such as greater Glasgow and Clyde, that experienced significant unemploy-ment with no hope of finding employment, coupled with an increase in income inequalities. This was accompanied by a significant reduction (a "cost-saving measure," or austerity) in funds to help prevent and treat drug use and provide support services.[81]

Many members of the white urban and suburban working and middle class in the United States, where addiction to opioids is rampant today, saw the American dream die for them in front of their very eyes. Manufacturing industries that provided the backbone for the dream left long ago for cheaper pastures abroad. The actual government-supported white cultural expecta-tions were eroding—fertilizing the ground for hopelessness to sprout.

But, there is another element to consider—political power plays. You may remember from earlier in this little history that when the Emperor Yongzheng of the Qing dynasty was concerned about the emerging power of political opposition, he first attempted to associate *madak,* the tobacco-opium-herb concoction favored by those heretics from the coast of Fujian, with immorality, danger, subversion, and rebellion. And second, when con-cerns escalated, he decreed complete prohibition of *madak.*

With that in mind, let's briefly look at one example from the social experience in the United States. When Nixon co-opted the War on Drugs (which had been ongoing for years, since the end of alcohol prohibition), it was a political play to diminish the power of the burgeoning antiwar forces in direct opposition to Vietnam. The administration also hoped to counter the legislative muscle of African Americans that had emerged with the passing of the Civil Rights Act of 1964. Consider the answer when journalist and writer Dan Baum asked Nixon's Counsel to the President for Domestic Affairs John Ehrlichman: "How did the United States entangle itself in a policy of drug prohibition that has yielded so much misery and so few good results?" Ehrlichman answered:

> The Nixon campaign in 1968, and the Nixon White House after that, had two enemies: the antiwar left and black people. You understand what I'm saying? We knew we couldn't make it illegal to be either against the war or black, but by getting the public to associate the hippies with marijuana and blacks with heroin, and then criminalizing both heavily, we could disrupt those communities. We could arrest their leaders, raid their homes, break up their meetings, and vilify them night after night on the evening news. Did we know we were lying about the drugs? Of course we did.[82]

Under the umbrella of preventing and fighting drug abuse and addiction, every president and both political parties since have maintained this policy. And, despite minimal differences in usage rates, minorities are significantly and disproportionally more often arrested and serve longer sentences than Caucasians.[83]

In the 1960s and 1970s, when it was mostly hippies and brown and black people using drugs for the exploration of consciousness, to self-medicate, or both, policies of enforcement were maintained without much question on the part of the greater public. However, now, the opioid addiction is affecting mostly white working-class people in the rural and suburban heartland of America. And, for the first time in decades, there seems to be a shift in the narrative. While before it was an iron-fist approach, today the new "white drug war" is framed in a significantly different color and context, calling for more understanding of the disease of addiction, for a more compassionate treatment-based approach—all the while keeping in place the iron-fist policies for people of color.[84]

The resulting cognitive dissonance stands as a red-alert beacon for all to sense and see. I've digressed slightly, but it's all important. Chapter 8 goes into more detail about the vulnerabilities that may contribute to addiction and what can be done in defense. This brief section about the modern epidemic was introduced primarily to show its parallels with popular use of opioids in other places and recent times.

Modern Applications and Modern Problems

> *If the entire materia medica at our disposal were limited to the choice and use of only one drug, I am sure that a great many, if not the majority, of us would choose opium; and I am convinced that if we were to select, say, half a dozen of the most important drugs in the Pharmacopeia, we should all place opium in the first rank.*
>
> —DAVID I. MACHT, MD[85]

While new and related opioid-based compounds have appeared regularly, morphine remains the standard of analgesia in the treatment of acute pain, such as postsurgery, against which all others are compared.

Methadone is one of the opioids that appeared and stayed. It was first developed by researchers at IG Farben (now Bayer) just before the outbreak of World War II. Shortly after the war ended, it was introduced to the United States for its primary use in the treatment of opioid dependence. Methadone, while potentially addictive by itself, helps reduce physical symptoms of opioid withdrawal, prolongs episodes of satiation, reduces opioid cravings, and produces some analgesic and antitussive effects, but with less pronounced sedation, and most importantly, less respiratory depression than morphine. One patient of mine compared methadone to heroin but without the fun.

The early 1960s brought us the synthetic opioids, starting with fentanyl, which is about eighty times the strength of morphine,[86] paling in comparison with the opioids appearing in the 1970s. These fentanyl analogs such as carfentanil (1974) are about 10,000 times stronger than morphine.[87]

CRUDE ESTIMATED STRENGTHS COMPARED
TO 10 MG MORPHINE (MS) INTRAVENOUSLY (IV)

OPIOIDS	× THE RELATIVE STRENGTH
(nonopioid-based analgesic) aspirin	0.003×
(nonopioid-based analgesic) ibuprofen	0.005×
codeine p.o. (orally)	0.05×
tapentadol	0.1×
opium (orally)	0.1×
morphine p.o.	0.3×
oxycodone p.o.	0.5×
morphine intravenously (10 mg = 1)	1
methadone (acute p.o.)	1×
oxycodone	2×
heroin (IV)	2–5×
buprenorphine (IV)	25×
fentanyl	50–100×[88]
carfentanil or lofentanil	10,000×[89]

And while physicians through time have individually learned about the appropriate use of opioids by observation, trial, and error, until roughly the 1970s nobody really knew how opioids worked inside the human body to realize their analgesic and other effects. That is until Candace Pert, who would later write the book *Molecules of Emotion,* and Solomon Snyder discovered the first opioid receptor site (mu, or μ) in mammalian tissue in 1973.[90]

It followed that if the human body makes opioid receptors, the body must make key-like molecules that fit into the receptors. A year later, two teams, one Scottish and the other from the United States, were credited with discovering the first such keys—endorphins (endogenous opioid neuropeptides), which were named by combining the Greek *endo-,* "from within," and the word *morphine.*[91] Endorphins are the brain's own opium, capable of reducing pain perception and stress, and instilling euphoria.[92] Five groups of endogenous opioids have so far been revealed: beta-endorphins, enkephalins, dynorphins, endomorphins, and nociceptin.[93]

In one of life's miracles, nature offers plants that can bind with the same receptor sites as our own, and provide us with stronger and longer-lasting euphoria and pain relief. Since the first discovery, numerous other opioid receptors have been identified and divided into four subtypes: the three classical types mu (μ), delta (δ), and kappa (κ), located in the brain, spinal cord, and gastrointestinal tract—these are primarily associated with inducing analgesic effects. The fourth type is the nociceptin (NOP) receptor, which has been shown either to have very low analgesic properties[94] or possibly to produce hyperalgesic effects (making pain sensation worse).[95]

The effectiveness of an opioid is dependent on a number of variables of the pain experience, such as location (central or peripheral), type of pain (acute or chronic), underlying causes (nociceptive, inflammatory, pathological), mental-emotional pain, gender, type of opioids used, and the presence, concentration, and type of opioid receptor in the location of pain. With all the progress made in modern times toward understanding the mechanism of pain, the analgesic properties, and potentially addicting properties of opioids, we still have much to learn.[96]

The Powers of Opioids:
The Good, the Bad, and the Ugly

Regardless of our current knowledge limitations, today opioids are essential life-saving drugs used in the field by paramedics and combat medics in the treatment of fractures, acute injuries, burns, acute pulmonary edema, or severe pains during a heart attack, among others. Beyond an emergency setting, opioids are often essential in the treatment of postsurgery pains, labor pains, certain chronic pains, intractable cancer pains, cough suppression, difficult-to-treat diarrhea, anesthesia, sedation, and opioid substitution therapy during opioid withdrawals (a.k.a. de-addiction), including dysphoric (mental discomfort) symptoms such as anxiety and depression.

Opioids are also employed in certain patients with sepsis or those who are critically ill, such as intensive care unit patients. However, indications under such circumstances are poorly understood, especially regarding the impact of opioids on hemodynamic and inflammatory counterresponses in cases of heart attack, blood loss, infection, and inflammation.

After reviewing the blessing that opioids can bestow, it is helpful to balance the picture and define its potential liabilities. Following is a list of opioids' common therapeutic, adverse, and deadly effects. Most of the items on the list are self-explanatory, while some, marked with an asterisk, are explained below.

OPIOIDS: SUMMARY EFFECTS CHART

Opioid-based analgesics include:	EFFECTS	
	Therapeutic Effects	
Vicodin	euphoria	yes
OxyContin	feeling "high"	yes
oxycodone	May be similar among opium, morphine, heroin, and different from other pharma-based opioids such as methadone or carfentanil, for example. Subjective experience depends on the route (smoked, nasal, ingested, injected, topical, suppository), concentration, and constitution of the user.	The opium, morphine, heroin high is often described as orgasmic but longer lasting, giving way to pleasure, sedation, relaxation, analgesia, and a sleepy-dream-like state void of any pain, fear, worry, or stress. Methadone is described as the high of heroin but without the fun.
hydrocodone		
fentanyl		
carfentanil		
codeine		
Demerol		
Percodan		
morphine		
heroin (the street version of morphine with about twice its strength)		
	sedation	yes
Opioid-based drugs for opioid withdrawal symptoms:	relaxation	yes
methadone	analgesia	yes
Opioid-based agonist-antagonist combination drugs for opioid withdrawal symptoms:	**Adverse Effects**	
	dysphoria (anxiety, depression)	yes
	sweating	yes
pentazocine	respiratory depression	yes
nalbuphine		
butorphanol	increased heart rate	yes
	hypotension (low blood pressure)	yes

EFFECTS	
Adverse Effects	
dry mouth	yes
constipation	yes
constricted pupils	yes
itching (pruritis)	yes
nausea/vomiting	yes
appetite	loss of
hyperalgesia	yes
addiction	high risk in some people; see chapter 8
physical withdrawal symptoms	yes
emotional blunting*	yes
reduction of empathy*	possible in certain people
reduced sex drive*	yes, with chronic use
reduced estrogen	yes
reduced testosterone	yes
serotonin syndrome*	yes
adrenal insufficiency*	yes
Deadly Effects	
respiratory arrest	yes
death due to fatal overdose	yes
increase risk of death due to infection	yes

Opioid use inhibits physical pain but may also cause **emotional blunting** of the affective component of pain[97] and imbalances in the endocrine system (endocrinopathy).[98] Consider a study conducted by Finnish researchers on the medical prescription history of 959 convicted murderers, which revealed that an increased risk of committing murder was not, as expected, creating spikes in people using antipsychotic medications, but in those under the influence of pain medications (opioid, nonopioid) and benzodiazepines.[99] In direct contrast, another study examining the effects of medical marijuana legalization (MML) on murder rates based on data from states with MML between 1990 and 2006 revealed a drop in homicides, rape, as well as other violent crimes in general.[100] Furthermore, as early as 1970, a researcher noted that the cannabis experience enhances empathy, connection, and insight, which would contribute to reductions in violent crime.[101]

Perhaps it should come as no surprise that a blunting or suppression of the flow of emotional material is also associated with stagnation or imbalance in the hormones, neurotransmitters, or other communication molecules normally associated with these emotions.

For instance, **serotonin syndrome** occurs when an overabundance of the neurotransmitter serotonin collects at the synapses; this can be caused by certain opioids (e.g., tramadol, meperidine, methadone).[102] And while symptoms range between mild and life-threatening, many times symptoms mirror that of opioid withdrawal, such as restlessness, tachycardia (rapid heartbeat), high blood pressure (hypertension), twitching, shivering, sweating, or diarrhea.[103]

As another example, emerging evidence suggests that chronic opioid use may weaken neurotransmitters or hormones produced by the adrenal glands, such as epinephrine and cortisol (responsible for fight, flight, and freeze reactions), leading to **adrenal insufficiency** or fatigue.[104] Chronic pharmaceutical use of opioids has also been linked to a **reduced sex drive** and a corresponding reduction in sex hormones.[105] Symptoms of decreased sex hormones (reduced testosterone and estrogen) include low libido in both genders, impotence, dysmenorrhea, and difficulties conceiving.[106] In contrast, you may recall the earlier mention of reports of opium used as an aphrodisiac. Obvious differences were cultural context and type of opioid used. This is something to ponder, since no study so far has examined the apparent paradox.

Defining Addiction

Addiction seems to be an inevitable part of the human condition; it is a cry for help in situations of suffering or grief.

—JEAN COCTEAU

While defining **addiction** seems at first glance trivial, the term is now omnipresent. For far too many, it is part of our daily lives. If not personal, it infuses its impact directly into the spheres of family or friends. If you are one of those lucky few who do not know anyone dealing with addiction, it is nonetheless a constant topic of discussion in the news and other media. The old models of addiction unfold on a spectrum ranging from one side asserting that the drug takes control and you are a victim, to the other extreme positing that addiction is a choice and only the feeble or weak-minded succumb, with theories such as self-medication landing somewhere in between.

Two of the most significant forces that drive opioid addiction are initial or ongoing pain and the pain of withdrawal or dysphoria (the term for the set of miserable physical and psychological symptoms that accompany termination of one's addictive substance). Logic dictates that before the appearance of withdrawal symptoms, there has to be the presence of addiction. Defining addiction itself, however, is notoriously difficult and has become an ongoing process as we learn more about the disease. While there are numerous aspects that have been illuminated in some way, nobody knows exactly what causes it. Nobody has the whole picture or a solution that works for everyone effectively and consistently. Continuing efforts to understand addiction involve investigation of a number of cultural, social, biological, psychological, and economic variables that can affect each person differently. However, addiction has a number of observable components that are practically recognized: There is the **high** or intoxication, or simply the cessation of pain. There is the notion of **reinforcement,** defined as "the drug's ability to make you want it once more." The concept of **tolerance** suggests that with each use, more has to be taken to achieve the same results. The experience of **dependence** refers to needing to use the drug even when faced with degenerating or destructive consequences. And, finally, there is the appearance of **withdrawal** symptoms when the drug is no longer taken.

From a clinical perspective, there is a distinction to be made between the use of drugs resulting in no harm (recreational, occasional, experimental), the abuse of drugs such as binge drinking (substance abuse), and the chronic, escalating use of drugs defined by loss of control over consumption despite evidence of harm, including the appearance of negative withdrawal symptoms in body, mind, and emotions that initiate and reinforce the cycle of addiction (substance dependence). The longer the cycle is active, the more intense and visible the deterioration. Generally, if using a substance is affecting someone's life, especially personal relationships, more negatively than positively, there is likely to be an addiction problem.

From a biological perspective, addiction is a neurological disease of the brain characterized by overpowering desire for the drug or other substances or even activities (sex, gambling, the internet) and a diminished ability to resist. A neuroscientist might look at addiction as involving those cellular and circuitry parts of the central nervous system that balance reward and stress or the seeking of pleasure and the avoidance of pain. In this context, for example, the key neurotransmitter system that is associated with the beginning of the cycle of addiction is dopamine—regulating reward-related mental and emotional expressions such as pleasure, cognition, emotion, and motivation. On the other hand, the neurotransmitter glutamate is associated with completing the cycle of addiction by promoting compulsivity and diminished control.[107]

A government perspective on addictive drugs has been enshrined and classified since 1961 by an international treaty called the Single Convention on Narcotic Drugs, which set the guidelines to control production and supply of a hundred or so drugs referred to as narcotics.[108] The term is derived from the ancient Greek word *narko,* meaning "to make numb," and it is actually not very well defined, but it is commonly used in legal contexts to delineate illicit drugs. For example:

Schedule I drugs are posited to have the highest potential of abuse (cannot be prescribed), hypothesized to have no medical value, and are generally considered unsafe. They include heroin (the only opioid in this category), LSD, ibogaine, cannabis, ecstasy (MDMA), and psilocybin.

Schedule II drugs are posited to have medical value (can be prescribed), believed to have a high potential for abuse, and include more opioids such as laudanum (opium) tincture, morphine, fentanyl, hydromorphone, methadone, and oxycodone. This schedule also lists amphetamines (speed), cocaine, barbiturates, and nabilone, a synthetic cannabinoid.

Schedule III drugs have a perceived potential for abuse and include the opioid buprenorphine, ketamine (an anesthetic), anabolic steroids such as testosterone, and the cannabinoid Marinol.

Schedule IV drugs have a perceived low potential for abuse and include benzodiazepines.

Schedule V drugs have the perceived lowest potential for abuse and include anticough medication containing small quantities of codeine.

Keep in mind that drugs on these lists were categorized almost sixty years ago by policy-makers influenced by a biased, ill-informed, prejudicial narrative straight out of the old propaganda movie *Reefer Madness* that reflects politically charged perceptions of perceived dangers. This narrative continues to receive well-deserved and significant criticism.

In addition to difficulties defining the specificity of addiction, it is challenging to establish a baseline to determine which drugs are most addictive or hazardous and as such should be prioritized in terms of risks and dangers. So, **what is the most addictive drug?** People would like to know. However, as you may have guessed by now, this is a very difficult question to answer because some people can take a drug for a long time and not get addicted, while some use it just a few times and experience significant problems with addiction. The difference? The presence of a great number of predisposing physical, psychological, and cultural conditions or vulnerabilities that play a significant role in developing drug dependence or addiction that can vary greatly among people. Thus the definition of addiction and the answer to which drug is most addictive largely depend on who you ask. The final chapter of this book will examine vulnerabilities and how to shore them up in greater detail.

Allow me to offer some context from my perspective as a former paramedic and as a current researcher. I used to judge the danger of a drug by the harmful impact it had on the people I treated and the frequency with which people needed to call 911 due to drug use. The number-one drug responsible for generating 911 emergency calls is nicotine contained in tobacco cigarettes, due to the lasting and serious damage that smoking causes, followed closely by alcohol abuse and sugar consumption–related mortality trends. Next came heroin, stimulants (cocaine, crack, methamphetamine, diet pills), and PCP.

You may notice the fact that drugs such as nicotine, alcohol, and sugar aren't even listed on any government schedule, while causing either directly or indirectly a significant and disproportional number of addiction-related 911 calls. In contrast, you may also notice the lack of 911 calls generated by drugs that are listed in Schedule I, such as cannabis, LSD, psilocybin, and ibogaine.

My work experience was echoed by research conducted by Daniel M. Perrine about the addictiveness of six commonly used substances. His results showed the most addictive drug to be nicotine, followed by alcohol, heroin, cocaine, caffeine, and lastly cannabis. You may want to take notice that according to these findings, alcohol is as addictive as heroin, and the most addictive substance, nicotine, is nowhere to be found on the government schedule. Meanwhile, Schedule I's cannabis was ranked the lowest for addiction potential by the Perrine study.[109]

Another large-scale survey conducted across the U.S. on more than eight thousand people ages fifteen to fifty-four described possible drug dependence patterns as follows: most prevalent was cigarettes, next was heroin. Cocaine and alcohol followed, and cannabis ranked among the lowest.[110] Whatever definition we might gravitate toward, the truth is that the exact cause or causes of addiction as well as its precise mechanism are still topics of considerable debate and the focus of ongoing research and scientific inquiry.

In contrast to the amorphous nature of definitions and approaches to drugs and addiction, the nature of opioid withdrawal symptoms is easily observable and clearly defined. Opioid withdrawal symptoms can be grouped roughly as follows:

General physical withdrawal symptoms: muscle cramps • involuntary movements • flu-like symptoms, fever, and chills • joint pain • increased sensitivity to pain • insomnia • fatigue

Gastrointestinal withdrawal symptoms: abdominal cramps and pains • diarrhea • nausea and vomiting • lack of appetite

Autonomic nervous system withdrawal symptoms: tachycardia • hypertension • runny nose • teary eyes • coryza (mucus build-up) • sweating • frequent yawning

Mental-emotional withdrawal symptoms: intense craving for opioids • restlessness • anxiety • dysphoria (opposite of euphoria) • increased stress, including low stress tolerance • depression

Orthodox medicine recognizes opioid use disorder[111] and opioid withdrawal[112] as an illness that is defined by diagnosis based on the guidelines of the *Diagnostic and Statistical Manual.* Most physicians use a pharmaceutical approach to managing symptoms with drugs such as methadone, buprenorphine, or naltrexone. A psychiatrist might combine a pharmaceutical approach with behavioral therapies, which are available to those with sufficient funds or a rare insurance carrier that provides for it. In-patient rehabilitation centers may offer a more complex number of services, such one-on-one talk therapy or group therapy addressing contributing factors to developing vulnerabilities for addiction and relapse tendencies, but these centers tend to be expensive and for now are out of reach for many in the United States. A free approach or twelve-step program is offered by organizations that adopted the Alcoholics Anonymous (AA) model of addiction and created an AA chapter for opioid users.

Jean Cocteau said, "But opium, the 'living substance,' like all drugs, exacts its price: the opium-eater is himself eaten by opium."[113] Studies show that between 1998 and 1999, nearly half of all heroin users (48 percent) in San Francisco had experienced a near-fatal overdose in their lifetime.[114] By 2016 the actual opioid overdose deaths in the United States had reached a staggering 53,332 lives lost.[115]

three

Cannabis, the Endocannabinoid System, and Pain: A Brief Overview

The Good, the Great, and the Concerns

ANCIENT ALLIES, PRESENT FRIENDS. The opium poppy flower, cannabis, and humanity have been inseparably linked ever since the first primordial opioid and cannabinoid receptors evolved 450 million and 600 million years ago, respectively.[116] Human DNA has continued to code for receptors that perfectly fit with both plants' key constituents. Chance, evolution, or divine intervention? However you look at it, it's fun to imagine how early humans discovered and learned to use the body- and mind-altering properties of both plants for purposes not dissimilar to our own, living here and now.

After exploring opium poppy complexities in detail in the previous chapter, let's now turn our attention to cannabis, whose history of medicinal and entheogenic* uses similarly dates back thousands of years. Cannabis was used in all medical traditions of the world, ancient and modern. And while its abundant healing capacities have long been a blessing to humankind, it wasn't until discovery of one of its key constituents, tetrahydrocannabinol (THC),

---

* After the Greek words *entheos,* "inspired by god," and *genesthai,* "to become," combined to mean "to inspire the divine within."

and the subsequent discovery of the first cannabinoid receptor and matching endogenous ligands (the body's own cannabinoids) that researchers could finally start to explain how the plant actually realizes its therapeutic potentials.

More specifically, this revolution in understanding started in 1963 when Raphael Mechoulam and Yehiel Gaoni were able to isolate Δ^9-tetrahydrocannabinol, or THC for short,[117] the primary and most studied constituent of cannabis, and the primary psychoactive component. The next "aha" moment came in 1990 when researchers from St. Louis University Medical School documented the first receptor, later named cannabinoid receptor 1 (or CB1), that binds with cannabis-based constituents.[118] Three years later, British scientists found a second receptor, CB2.[119]

The next puzzle piece marked another critical point in the emerging cannabinoid health sciences. Once more, it was Mechoulam and team who brought forth the characterization of the first endogenous cannabinoid.[120] *Endo-* is from the Greek word for "within," and *cannabinoid* comes from the name *cannabis.* In other words, the world became privy to the fact that the body makes its own version of THC.

Mechoulam and his team named the compound "anandamide" by combining the Sanskrit word for "bliss," *ananda,* and the scientific word *amide,* describing an organic chemical compound. Of the handful of endocannabinoids discovered today, the most significant regarding the potential for therapeutic impact in terms of analgesia and opioid withdrawal symptoms is anandamide, "the bliss molecule."

Once the foundational pieces of the puzzle were in place, a growing number of scientists quickly realized that throughout the human body, present in all organ systems, exists a vast network of cannabinoid receptors and endocannabinoids. These molecules made by the human body operate together, much like locks and keys. When a connection is made, receptors are unlocked, and complex sets of physical, mental, and emotional responses that are therapeutically relevant to pain quickly unfold. The entire system was named the endocannabinoid system (ECS).

Cannabinoids come in three forms: those made inside and by the human body (endocannabinoids); those from the outside (exocannabinoids) made by plants, primarily cannabis (called phytocannabinoids); and artificial (synthetic) cannabinoids.

While scientific progress was made, and while the successful albeit still illicit uses of cannabis in cases of people dying from cancer or suffering from complications of a chronic disease were noticed by the orthodox medical community, there was still no practical information available with which to scientifically discern the age-old anecdotally therapeutic benefits of the plant, especially in cases of chronic conditions and stubborn symptoms—one of which is pain.

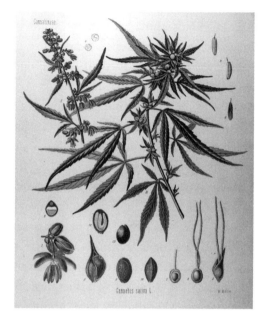

Pain is mitigated by changes realized in body, mind, or emotions. Analgesic effects occur in the body when we induce changes in the pain-processing centers of the brain, such as the amygdala, the insula, or the anterior cingulate cortex; to the circuitry of pain, including the relays between peripheral nerves, the spinal cord, the thalamus, the basal ganglia, and the cerebral cortex; or to the transmission of pain signals via numerous messenger molecules such as glutamate, GABA, epinephrine, and cortisol. Similarly, changes in cognition structures—our pain narrative, coping mechanisms, focus, and beliefs around pain—can downregulate sensitivity to pain and thereby mitigate the experience of pain. And finally, shifts in the biology of affect (emotions) can significantly alter pain perceptions: for example, feeling relaxed and safe can reduce pain perception.

Of the nearly 150 plant-based cannabinoids that have been identified to date, only a few tend to exist naturally in large enough concentrations to therapeutically affect pain perceptions in humans. Of those, the most significant are tetrahydrocannabinol (THC) and cannabidiol (CBD). The reader is advised that other cannabis-based constituents have been shown to provide effective analgesia, but due to the scope of this book, we will focus on those with the greatest and most established potential.

Similar to synthetic opioids (think carfentanil), synthetic or artificial cannabinoids tend to be isolated molecules that are many times more potent in the specific effects they produce than their very distant natural cousins. They are also void of the synergy and balance-building properties of natural, full-spectrum cannabis.[121] Therefore, a more appropriate discernment would be to compare them with pharmaceuticals that are associated with potential severe adverse reactions. Synthetic cannabinoids have their place in research and may even have some safe and effective therapeutic application yet to be determined. The most common synthetic cannabinoids are the following (in alphabetical order, with x standing for various numbers): 5F-x, AM-x, CP-x, JWH-x, HU-x, O-x, SR-x, WIN-x. You may come across news reports talking of the significant dangers associated with "spice" or other synthetic cannabinoids easily obtained on the internet. It is these groups of chemicals that are referred to, and as such they deserve a brief mention.

Cannabinoid receptors are widely spread across numerous pain-modulating pathways, such as central and peripheral sensory neurons, brain regions modulating sensory discrimination, pain-regulatory circuitry in the brain stem, and affective states that regulate emotional responses to noxious stimuli.[122] The body's own endocannabinoids may provide one of the earliest therapeutic responses to pain[123] by unlocking one or more of the available pathways to realizing analgesic effects.

How Can Cannabis Relieve My Pain?

Cannabinoids—both those made by the human body and plant-based versions—have demonstrated the ability to bind to cannabinoid receptors and as such are uniquely positioned to mitigate pain in all its complexities. Thus speedy relief and, perhaps more importantly, deeper and more complete healing may be realized in virtually all cases of chronic, central, peripheral, nociceptive, inflammatory, pathological, and mental-emotional pain. However, the means and pathways by which cannabinoids realize analgesic effects are manifold but can be practically divided in those constituents that kill pain by getting you high and those that don't (see figures 3.1 and 3.2 below).

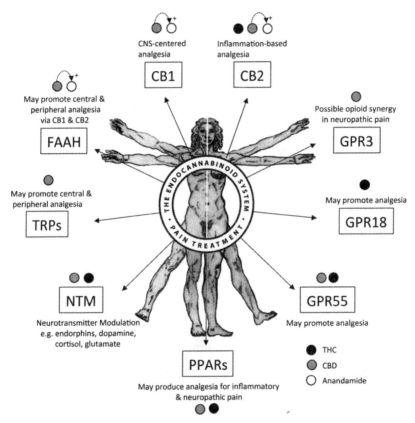

Figure 3.1. Nonpsychoactive (THC, CBD, and anandamide-based) pathways relevant to pain and analgesia

Anandamide fits relatively equally into both CB1 and CB2 receptors (the "locks"), and activation of these receptors can modulate processes such as pain, addiction, and withdrawal via these and other receptors,[124] but at about a tenth of the strength of THC at CB1, and about one-thirteenth the strength of THC at CB2.[125] Once a connection is made, the lock opens and a signal is generated. At that point, numerous physiological as well as mental and emotional changes take place. In general, anandamide initiates a host of changes in both the central nervous system (CNS, consisting of the brain and spinal cord), primarily via CB1, and the immune system, primarily via CB2, as well as the autonomic nervous system (ANS) with its two subdivisions of parasympathetic (downer effect, feed and breed, rest and digest) and sympathetic (upper effect, fight or flight or freeze). Some specific examples suggest that anandamide may reduce the sensation of pain in the periphery[126] and may mitigate neuropathies[127] and inflammation-based pains.[128]

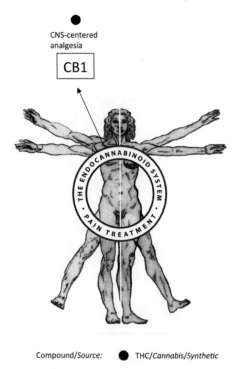

CNS-centered analgesia

CB1

Compound/Source: ● THC/Cannabis/Synthetic

Figure 3.2. The primary (THC-based) psycho-active pathway relevant to pain and analgesia

Research conducted on mice discovered that after anandamide was injected, the compound moved through different tissues at different rates. For instance, while brain peak levels occurred around the five-minute mark, the endogenous cannabinoid was quickly metabolized there with no detectable levels after fifteen minutes. However, fifteen minutes after administration, the general analgesic effects were still at 85 percent of maximum, suggesting the possibility that anandamide initiated the release of other compounds that produce analgesic effects.[129] Anandamide is degraded by the enzyme fatty acid amide hydrolase (FAAH), and lower levels of FAAH increase the bioavailability of anandamide, which in turn can induce analgesic effects via CB1 and CB2, as described above.[130]

This brings us to cannabis-based constituents CBD and THC, which similarly bind with a number of receptors that open pathways to initiate painkilling effects in body, mind, and emotions. Properly used for an individual's specific constitution and needs, cannabis is a promising therapy for a wide range of conditions, including the chronic pain for which opioids are so often used and the misery of opioid withdrawal. However, as many patients have discovered, once you find the product that works for you—be it smoking, vaporizing, consuming cannabis cookies or chocolate, or taking a tincture—it can become a simple and safe process that does provide pain relief. Patients, doctors, and research scientists continue to work out details, with or without the support of the U.S. federal government. The information in this book is a start toward understanding the science and the possibilities, while much remains to be solidified in practice.

Cannabidiol (CBD) is a nonpsychoactive cannabinoid with the capacity for positively influencing affectual (emotional) states of mind via modulation of various neurotransmitters, and as such CBD can shift dysphoria associated with pain and withdrawal.[131] For instance, CBD initiates activation of serotonin (5-HT$_{1A}$) receptors[132] and thus lowers heart rate,[133] produces mood improvements,[134] and aids arousal.[135] While CBD has little direct affinity for either CB1 or CB2,[136] some of its therapeutic influence stems from its ability to suppress the enzyme fatty acid amide hydrolase (FAAH), keeping the "bliss molecule" active at higher concentrations and for a longer duration, thus indirectly, naturally, and "gently" activating CB1- and CB2-initiated effects.[137]

CBD is considered a very promising agent in the cotreatment of pain in conjunction with opioids. It can boost opioid-based analgesic effects, allowing for lower doses that are effective, while reducing the risk of addiction and overdose. For instance, German researchers discovered in rodent experiments that both CBD and to a lesser degree THC (six times less than CBD) bind noncompetitively with mu (μ) and delta (δ) opioid receptors[138] and thus may potentially enhance the effects of opioids. If confirmed in humans, this synergy could explain why many patients using opioids for the treatment of pain tend to use significantly less when also medicating with cannabis.

Because CBD has been found to be capable of protecting nerves from damage,[139] it can potentially mitigate numerous underlying mechanisms involved in various types of pain and withdrawal, such as oxidative stress. In addition, CBD has been shown to bind to receptors other than the classical cannabinoid receptors CB1 and CB2 in the context of pain and withdrawal. For example, CBD binds to TRPA1 receptors,[140] which are relevant to pain, itching, and inflammation. It also binds with TRPV1 receptors[141] and produces analgesic effects, especially in inflammation.[142] And lastly, CBD may initiate analgesic effects in cases of inflammation and neuropathic pains via peroxisome proliferator-activated receptors (PPARs, pronounced "peepars").[143]

Delta-9-tetrahydrocannabinol (THC) is the primary mind-altering constituent of cannabis and is responsible for generating complex changes in body, mind, and emotion.[144] Like anandamide, THC binds relatively equally with both CB1 and CB2 receptors but in a stronger fashion, producing more intense and longer-lasting effects. Numerous preclinical and clinical trials have demonstrated THC's primary analgesic and psychotropic effect to be mediated via CB1 receptors,[145] while inflammation-based pains were found to be mitigated by THC's activation of CB2 receptor sites.[146] And, perhaps more practically relevant, recent trials conducted on humans demonstrated THC's analgesic efficacy in cases of chronic pains.[147] Beyond inducing analgesic effects via the classical G-protein-coupled receptors CB1 and CB2, THC may also produce pain relief by binding with other members of the super family of G-protein-coupled receptors, namely GPR18[148] and GPR55.[149]

THC has been shown to induce analgesic effects by modulating a great variety of neurotransmitters relevant to the transmission of pain, such as endogenous opioids. Indirect and noncompetitive binding at opioid receptor sites may also induce analgesic effects and as such provide a coadministered synergy with a number of potential benefits, such as boosting opioid-based analgesia at a lower dose.[150] THC may also initiate pain-reducing effects at ionotropic cannabinoid receptor sites relevant to heat, cold, itching, and inflammation-based pains.[151] Additional analgesia is realized via neurotransmitter modulation such as serotonin or acetylcholine pathways. (For more information about THC's capacity to modulate other neurotransmitters, see chapter 6.)

And similarly to CBD, THC may produce analgesic effects in cases of inflammation-based and neuropathic pains via PPARs. Figure 3.2 on page 44 represents the primary psychotropic THC-based pathway relevant to pain and analgesia.

What Are the Basic Types of Cannabis and Their Relevance for Pain and Opioid Withdrawal?

When we consider a pharmaceutical solution to mitigate pain, most people understand that while Vicodin, Xanax, and Ativan are all pills, they can't be taken expecting the same results. They are in fact different products with uniquely different chemical makeups and thus will produce very different effects: Vicodin for pain, Xanax for anxiety, and Ambien for sleep.

However, many people make the mistake of assuming that all cannabis is the same. This is not so. Cannabis or cannabinoid-containing products can vary greatly in the composition of biologically active constituents, and as such can induce very different effects. Knowing what cannabis type produces what effect goes a long way toward achieving the analgesia you want.

For instance, did you know that one of three type of cannabis will create a significant synergy with opioids and gently uplift your emotions, but without any changes in cognition (without getting you "high")? Learning the basic distinctions allows you to make more informed decisions about which cannabis type may be the best option for you to produce the symptom reductions, improvements in mood, or well-being you are looking for. It also greatly determines your ability to do it safely and to sustain the desired effects while reducing the risk of unwanted effects.

You may also want to think of these cannabis **chemotypes** as your unique cannabis prescription that are informed by the currently available scientific evidence.

In 1973, the researchers E. Small and H. D. Beckstead devised a system of classification of individual cannabis plants[152] that continues to inform the emerging cannabinoid health sciences of today. It's a ratio-based system focusing on the volume of THC and CBD, the most abundant cannabinoids found in cannabis. Each plant can be assigned to one of three discrete chemotypes designated by the Roman numerals I, II, and III. In a nutshell: **Chemotype I** contains more THC than CBD. **Chemotype II** contains relatively equal amounts of THC to CBD, close to 1:1. **Chemotype III** contains more CBD than THC, or no THC at all.[153]

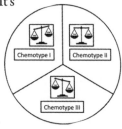

Two additional chemotypes were tentatively reported in the scientific literature: chemotypes IV and V. Neither contributes unique, practical, or therapeutically significant information that is not already covered by chemotypes I through III, or by reports on the biological impact of individual cannabinoids. Chemotype IV reported by Fournier et al. in 1987[154] was defined as having CBG as the most abundant cannabinoid. Chemotype V proposed by Mandolino and Carboni in 2004[155] includes strains that are void of any detectable cannabinoids.

⚖️ Chemotype I

A pharmaceutical example of a chemotype I–based product would be dronabinol, a synthetic or chemical version of THC. To apply the ratio concept, it would be represented as THC:CBD (1:0). A double-blind placebo-controlled trial discovered similar analgesic effects between dronabinol (10 or 20 mg) compared to smoking a low-concentration cannabis (~2 percent or ~3.5 percent THC). Adverse effects were a slight increase in heart rate with both smoked cannabis and ingested THC compared to placebo.[156] Another relevant double-blind, placebo-controlled trial conducted on patients suffering from chronic pains who use opioids discovered that synthetic THC (dronabinol) produced additional synergistic analgesic effects.[157] An additional placebo-controlled experiment conducted on twenty opioid-dependent individuals concluded that dronabinol was able to reduce the severity of opiate withdrawal symptoms during the acute phase of the detoxification process.[158]

To date in the United States, the FDA allows the marketing of dronabinol for the treatment of anorexia (appetite stimulation) associated with weight loss in patients with HIV/AIDS and as an antiemetic in chemotherapy-induced nausea and vomiting. Adverse effects of dronabinol may include: euphoria ("feeling high"), altered consciousness, paranoia, anxiety, increased heart rates, insomnia, pain, or nausea.

The top chemotype I cannabis flowers that were laboratory tested in 2016 included strains such as: Godfather OG (~34 percent THC)[159], Super Glue (~32 percent THC)[160], and Strawberry Banana (~32 percent THC).[161] No information was given regarding CBD content. Adverse effects of chemotype I strains may include those listed for dronabinol above. The reader is reminded that while "feeling high"—experiencing altered consciousness, or extraordinary states of awareness—may be considered by some an adverse effect, these symptoms can also be sought after by others for therapeutic, creative, or transpersonal purposes. Most adverse effects can be managed by reassurance and being in a safe, calm, relaxing atmosphere. Playing gentle music or nature sounds, holding hands if desired, or just being there can make the difference.

WHAT IS "GETTING HIGH"?

Getting "high" means experiencing widespread effects on cognitive functions such as enhancement and sharpness of the senses; shifts in perception of time, space, and the things in it; loss of short-term memory; changes in patterns of normal emotional responses or impulses (e.g., "normally I get angry when you push my buttons, but now I just feel at ease and relaxed with a sense of compassion for you and myself"; or "This is incredibly funny"). Getting high also refers to possible changes in motor function such as slower response times, unsteady gait (ataxia), or differences in speech patterns.

Sound weird? Do you wonder why people do it? Effects vary for individuals, but in general, many people find that the general muscle relaxation induced by cannabis extends to a mental shift toward relaxing—letting go, if only temporarily, of stress, worry, old rutted patterns of thought, annoyance, even anger. Usual mental loops are replaced by more novel thoughts and feelings, somewhat like flipping a toggle switch in your mind. A good cannabis experience can be compared to when the beauty and wholeness of nature or a child's love and enthusiasm wash over you and remind you what is really important in life. The superficial worries lose their consuming grip on you. This can provide relief from mental anguish, pain, or compulsion; or it may lead to creative insights as one views an art project or home-improvement task in a completely different way. The unique ability of cannabis to open up new ways of thinking is a particularly valuable asset when overcoming addiction and all its mental and emotional methods of attaching to the experience of substance use, need, and desire. Cannabis is well known to "shift the energy" of a range of problems, issues, feelings, and physical pains, but science is still catching up with what individuals only know as relief, getting high, loosening up, or a hundred other idioms for *feeling better.*

However, it's also possible that using cannabis (or the wrong chemotype for you) ratchets up innate tendencies for hyperactive, stressed-out, or paranoid thoughts and actions. If you aren't familiar with its effects in you, cautious experimentation is warranted. Cannabinoids can create different responses in different individuals. Getting high can be great or not great at all—there is definitely a range of possible experiences. Give yourself the benefit of a learning curve if you are new to cannabis use. Of course, if you've been taking opioids for a while, you are no stranger to physical and mental alterations and deviations from "normal" … you will find that the high differs, however.

⚖️ *Chemotype II*

Chemotype-II strains may provide the user with the synergy and balance-building properties of both of the plant's prime constituents, THC and CBD.[162] The primary group to benefit from a chemotype II includes patients who need central nervous system activation but in a more moderate or tempered version (compared to chemotype-I strains). By balancing the ratio of THC to CBD to near one to one, patients still receive modulation in and between CNS, mind, and mood, while CBD calms and potentially reduces the otherwise more powerful effects of THC on the mind—thereby reducing the risk of unwanted effects on perception, cognition, or mood such as extraordinary states of consciousness, strange ways of thinking, or uncontrollable euphoria, paranoia, or depression, which may occur in susceptible individuals using a chemotype I. Patients who tend to benefit from a chemotype II include those suffering from pain, such as neuropathic pain and fibromyalgia, and mental-emotional pain such as dysphoria, anxiety, and depression.

A popular pharmaceutical version of a chemotype II-based product is the oromucosal spray Sativex, extracted from whole-plant cannabis with a ratio of ~1:1 of its prime constituents THC and CBD. Sativex has been approved in the United Kingdom for the treatment of neuropathic pains and spasticity. Regarding its effectiveness as a painkiller, consider that a double-blind, placebo-controlled trial conducted on 263 opioid-treated cancer patients with intractable pain discovered that Sativex may be a useful add-on analgesic for this patient population.[163] The results were confirmed by a review of seven other placebo-controlled trials, six of which demonstrated positive analgesic effects.[164]

Adverse effects of Sativex may include: dizziness or fatigue (very common); dry mouth, disorientation, depression (common); throat irritation or application irritation; feeling high; and rapid heart rate (uncommon).[165]

The top chemotype II cannabis flowers that were laboratory tested in 2016 included strains such as: Cellar CBD, ~7.3% THC to ~7.7% CBD;[166] and Nubia, ~8% THC to ~7.5% CBD;[167] Hayley's Comet, with THC less than 15% and CBD more than 10%.[168] A local grower here in Berkeley, California, just came in at ~11%[169] THC and CBD for a chemotype-II called LT

Fire (*L* for Jamaican Lion and *T* for Purple Tabernacle, the parent strains). Adverse effects of chemotype-II strains may include dizziness, dry mucous membranes (mouth), and disorientation.

⚖ *Chemotype III*

Any cannabis flower or THC- and CBD-containing product that is composed of more CBD than THC is part this chemotype. Cannabis-using patients who tend to choose and benefit from a chemotype III include those in need of a general uplift in mood but who do not want to experience a "high" effect. Patients who seek to boost opioid-based analgesic effects, patients with neurological conditions such as various spasmotic or seizure disorders, those with opioid dependencies, or those dealing with dysphoria-related issues such as depression, anxieties, or psychotic disorders may prefer a chemotype-III cannabis medicine.

Mental and emotional effects at the positive end of the spectrum include a gentle uplift in mood with no effects on cognitive abilities. Thinking, perception, and sensory experiences remain unaltered. However, in some sensitive patients, use of a chemotype III that contains a significant level of THC may still produce adverse effects such as anxiety, although in much milder forms when compared to high-THC chemotype I.

A pharmaceutical example of chemotype III would be Epidiolex, a plant-derived cannabidiol-only medication with a THC:CBD ratio of 0:1.[170] Treatment examples from various countries where Epidiolex is legal include treatment-resistant epilepsy syndromes such as Dravet syndrome, Lennox-Gastaut syndrome, tuberous sclerosis complex, and infantile spasms.[171] Strain examples include Cannatonic, CBD OG, AC/DC, and Charlotte's Web.

Chemotype-III strains that have no, negligible, or relatively low amounts of THC are generally considered safe in humans, including for chronic use and high doses, up to 1,500 mg/day.[172] However, in terms of potential adverse effects, some studies have discovered that CBD may interfere with some pharmaceutical drugs metabolized by the liver.[173] Furthermore, CBD-only chemotype III may produce pro- and anti-inflammatory responses, and as such can reduce inflammation in many patients or increase inflammation in certain severely immunocompromised patients.[174] As you perhaps expected, the treatment indications as well as adverse effects for the pharmaceutical versions and corresponding strains tend to mirror each other.

The choice of the chemotype of cannabis that is going to work best for you is a subjective process in part guided by your priorities, preferences, and needs, and whenever possible ought to include a discernment based on the current available scientific literature, including peer-informed trends. If, for example, you want to avoid any altered state in consciousness—you want to avoid getting high—you can start with a chemotype III, which is represented by the bottom slice of the pie chart in figure 3.3. If you wish to harness a synergy of THC and CBD, you may want to start in the middle with a chemotype II. And finally, if you want or need to harness specific THC-induced qualities and are prepared to constructively handle shifts in cognition (you have some prior experience with THC), you may want to consider starting with a chemotype I, on the left side of the graphic.

Cannabis: The Concerns

The bottom line is that extensive evidence indicates that cannabis is neither dangerous nor harmless. Consideration of its medicinal use should include a risk versus benefit analysis, focused on the specific therapeutic needs and health challenges of the individual in question. Both knowledge of and respect for the cannabis plant will improve the outcome of consumption, whatever your goal.

Safety: According to several U.S. government sources, there were zero deaths due to the exclusive use of cannabis in the period studied, which ranged from January 1997 through June 2005.[175] (Deaths in which cannabis was one of several drugs used are not counted here.) In contrast, recent estimates by the Centers for Disease Control suggest that, on average, tobacco (particularly cigarette smoking) claimed 443,000 lives per year from 2000 to 2004.[176] The number of alcohol-related fatalities was estimated at 75,766 in 2001.[177]

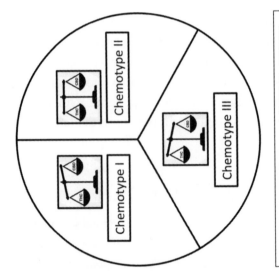

Top 3 Chemotype II Strains: LT Fire (THC ~ 11% and CBD ~11%), Cellar CBD (~7.3% THC to ~7.7% CBD), Nubia (~8% THC to ~7.5% CBD)

Popular Chemotype II Strains (alphabetically): CannaTsu, Hayley's Comet, One to One (OTO), Pennywise, Royal Highness, Rubicon, Stephen Hawking Kush, Sour Tsunami

Chemotype II Pharmaceutical Drug:
Sativex (each spray contains 2.7 mg THC and 2.5 mg CBD)

Top 3 Chemotype III Strains: Cannatonic (0.8% THC to 20.8% CBD), CBD OG (9.01% THC to 19.5% CBD), AC/DC (0.8% THC to 15.4% CBD)

Popular Chemotype III Strains (alphabetically): Avidekel, CBD Critical Cure, Cellar CBD, Charlotte's Web, Harlequin, HarleTsu, Nubia, Ringo's Gift, Tora Bora, Trident

Chemotype III Pharmaceutical Drug:
Epidiolex (98% oil-based CBD extract)(dose range ~5-20mg/kg/d)

Top 5 Chemotype I Strains: Godfather Og (~34% THC), Super Glue (~32% THC), Strawberry Banana (~32% THC), Venom OG Kush (~31% THC), Redeye Og (~30% THC)

Popular Chemotype I Strains (alphabetically): Blue Dream, Bruce Banner, Jack Herer, Girl Scout Cookies, Gorilla Glue, Grand Daddy Purple, Northern Lights, Og Kush, Sour Diesel

Chemotype I Pharmaceutical Drug:
Dronabinol (THC 2.5mg, 5mg, and 10mg soft gel capsules)

Figure 3.3. Examples of Cannabis Strains and Their Typical Chemotypes

Addiction potential: Opponents and proponents of medical cannabis both cite numerous studies to support their arguments for or against addiction, yet one distinction is usually agreed upon: if dependency occurs, it is an addiction in psychological terms rather than in the physical realm, while physical addiction is the case with many other substances, such as tobacco, alcohol, and heroin. The large numbers of people enrolled in drug treatment centers is often cited to substantiate claims that the cannabis plant is psychologically addictive. This overlooks the reality that many court judges do not believe cannabis users should go to jail, but as they are bound to uphold present laws, they are left with no other option but to mandate drug treatment instead of jail or prison time.

Compared to pharmaceuticals, some of which have a significant addiction potential, cannabis carries a greatly reduced risk of adverse side effects, including death. An FDA report compared cannabis to seventeen common FDA-approved pharmaceutical drugs used to treat similar symptoms and conditions. The findings make a compelling argument for medical cannabis. Between 1997 and 2005, no deaths were attributed to the exclusive use of cannabis, while the FDA recorded 10,008 deaths due to the seventeen FDA-approved pharmaceutical drugs in the study.[178]

If you are concerned about developing a dependence on cannabis, you may reduce this extremely low yet potential risk by choosing a cannabis flower with the chemotype III—meaning that it has a very high concentration of CBD and a very low concentration of THC. You may also choose from a variety of cannabis-containing ingestible products of the chemotype III variety. Ingestibles allow you to consume a CBD-only product void of any psychotropic effects. You may choose raw preparations of cannabis, which also have little or no psychoactive effect. Or, finally, you can choose a mindfulness technique to increase endocannabinoid presence and balance and thus get high on your body's own chemicals. For instance, recent studies suggest that the endocannabinoid system modulates the production and release of oxytocin.[179] Oxytocin, commonly referred to as the "cuddle molecule," is able to reduce pain[180] and promote wound healing[181] and is involved in the development of trust[182] and generosity.[183] To further reduce any risk of addiction, taking a break for a few days between treatments will serve this purpose, as well as help you avoid developing a tolerance.

Adverse effects: When it comes to fertility, the developing fetus, or the still physically developing adolescent, the use of any substances that can alter the mind or body is cause for concern. Various studies are cited by people on both sides of this issue as evidence for their position. No long-term studies examining the exclusive use of cannabis on fertility, the fetus, and adolescents have been conducted, with the exception of the Duke study discussed below. People enrolled in most studies of this nature are exposed to other substances, thus complicating the overall picture.

However, a study conducted at Duke University[184] that collected subjective observational data from New Zealand residents over a period of about thirty-eight years[185] concluded that while cannabis use by adults has no effect on intelligence, "cannabis dependency" in adolescents (defined by the authors as continued use despite major health, social or legal problems related to its use) may contribute to reduced IQ test scores later in life. This study has limitations: Data were described subjectively, the study had a small sample size (17 percent or 153 people met the authors' dependency definition), and only some factors that may alter IQ were considered in the analysis. This is the only study to date to examine the impact of adolescent use of cannabis on intelligence measured over time. Until more is known, it is advisable to assume a possible correlation.

Respiratory effects: Whenever plant matter is burned, smoke is released, and with it, potentially harmful particles. However, the largest population-based case-controlled study ever conducted of cannabis-only use yielded somewhat counterintuitive results. For the 2,252 people observed in a Los Angeles study, smoking only cannabis was found to be mildly lung-protective and was not associated with an increased risk of lung cancer.[186]

Cannabis oil produces therapeutic effects in patients with chronic obstructive pulmonary disease (a serious lung disorder)[187] and asthma.[188] To minimize any potential risk of negative consequences to one's lungs, some people use vaporizers to inhale cannabis rather than smoking cannabis wrapped in paper. Use of a vaporizer eliminates the inhalation of carbon compounds from burned paper. An infused oil or alcohol-based tincture can also be used to address symptoms related to lung diseases.

Cannabis and my heart: Endocannabinoid receptors are present in the heart and are involved in regulating heart function. THC can increase one's heart rate, but usually not to a dangerous extent. Furthermore, numerous studies have shown that THC and CBD as well as a variety of other cannabinoids have potentially potent cardioprotective properties.[189]

Cannabis and cancer: To date, no evidence supports the genesis of cancer due to cannabis consumption. In fact, numerous constituents of cannabis have demonstrated remarkable abilities to produce apoptosis (cancer cell death) in a great variety of cancer manifestations. Of course, any sort of smoking or even breathing air that is heavily laden with particulates may contribute to pulmonary stress.

Cannabis and psychosis: Observational studies have concluded that consuming cannabis as an adolescent may increase one's risk of developing schizophrenia later in life, particularly if there is an existing tendency. While cannabis is not itself a causal factor for schizophrenia, in some instances it may be a cofactor. Based on the current evidence, it would be prudent for adolescents or young adults with a known family history of psychosis or schizophrenia to stay away from cannabis or any other mind-altering substance, especially speed-based drugs such as cocaine or methamphetamine.

Is cannabis a "gateway drug"? The controversial gateway theory proposes that adolescents who experiment with cannabis are more likely to subsequently try, and become addicted to, other illicit drugs.[190] While the gateway theory has never attempted to address therapeutic uses of legally obtained medicine, the suggestion that even short-term cannabis use could lead to addiction to other drugs still lingers in many people's minds. Science as well as widespread anecdotal experience refute this association. In fact, a recent study of more than four thousand cannabis smokers concluded that cannabis use leads to a *decrease* in the use of alcohol, tobacco, and hard drugs.[191]

Can cannabis kill me? A laboratory study conducted in 1973 reported the median lethal dose of oral THC in rats to be 800–1,900 mg/kg, depending on the sex and genetic strain of the animal.[192] If body weight is used as the sole criteria, this study suggests that 200 grams of herb per kilogram of body weight are required to approach a lethal dose in humans. Accordingly, a person weighing 70 kilograms, or 154 pounds, would need to consume 14 kilograms of herb to approach a fatal dose. A 2004 study was much more conservative, stating "628 kilograms of cannabis would have to be smoked in 15 minutes to induce a lethal effect."[193]

four

Pain: Contrasting
Opioids and Cannabinoids
in Pain Management

THIS CHAPTER DISTINGUISHES AMONG different types of pain and discusses the usefulness of opioids, cannabis, and their combination in treating and managing pain, including mental-emotional pain. How to discover one's own specific cannabis chemotype prescription is described, so if you have never tried cannabis before, this chapter will introduce you to some basic information. Even if you have smoked cannabis for some time and consider yourself familiar with its effects, you are likely to learn something fresh about its distinctions and abilities from the new science that is emerging today.

Understanding Cannabis Prescriptions
Determining the Chemotype of Cannabis
Best Suited to Meet Your Needs and Preferences

Since specific cannabis constituents influence body, cognition, and affect in such a way as to induce physical relaxation, calmness of mind, analgesic effects, and an uplift in mood, even in the presence of otherwise emotionally difficult or intolerable experiences, they offer good prospects for producing deeper healing on every level of the human experience.

For example, Alzheimer's patients deal with cognitive decline such as loss of memory, emotional disorders such as irritability, and often experience chronic pains in combination. Now, recent clinical trials have shown that Alzheimer's patients respond especially well to cannabinoid-based therapies without the risks and costs of the regular cocktail of pharmaceuticals used in such cases.[194] There is one caveat: it greatly helps to know which kind of cannabis to use. Chapter 3 introduced this topic and the three chemotypes in more detail.

Let's summarize: The difference between the cannabis chemotypes is dependent on the ratio between THC and CBD. While both THC and CBD can produce analgesic effects, they do it by very different mechanisms. For instance, one of the ways THC produces analgesic effects is by binding with CB1 receptors in portions of the brain that also govern cognition, thus bringing a "high" effect. In contrast, CBD-based analgesia is produced via other mechanisms, such as indirectly binding with opioid receptor sites or by increasing the bioavailability of anandamide, which then binds with CB1 to produce analgesic effects, but at only about a tenth of the strength of THC, and void of psychotropic changes.[195]

A chemotype I always contains more THC than CBD, a chemotype II contains a relatively equal amount of both, while a chemotype III always contains more CBD than THC. The amount or concentration of THC determines the mind-altering effects. Figure 3.3 on page 54 was designed to visibly depict the chemotype range. The left slice (chemotype I) represents cannabis strains with the highest amount of THC, while the bottom slice represents strains with the highest amount of CBD and little to no THC, thus no mind-altering effects or high. Chemotype II is depicted by the slice of on the right side of the pie, with equal amounts of both cannabinoids.

One way to make more informed decisions about which cannabis chemotype will work best for you and the particular type of pain you are dealing with is to review the currently available literature; see the references at the back of this book, cited in the note numbers in the text. As you will see, in some cases there are clear trends that indicate a specific chemotype thought to work most efficaciously for a specific condition or type of pain: THC or CBD, in particular, is used to show associated effect demonstrated in the review. Other times, scientific evidence is underwhelming and subject to more interpretation. However, plenty of patients are experimenting with cannabis medicines on their own, and often their anecdotal stories are available online for reference and consideration.

In the absence of better trials, patients wanting to use cannabis or cannabis-containing products to treat pain may choose according to their preference regarding what type of cannabis experience they wish to have—and these choices will inevitably involve some trial and error. In other words, do you want to get really high or stoned in the process of relaxing that nagging pain, or just partially? If yes, then try more THC (chemotype I). If you want to gently experiment with pain relief, such as reducing inflammation and chronic pains[196] or picking up your mood, start with the "weaker" strains that are low in THC and unlikely to overwhelm you with "high" symptoms. In this case, seek cannabis types that are rich in CBD (chemotype III).

You may find it helpful to go look at Figure 4.1 and fill out the check boxes to see which chemotype is a match for you.

For each type of pain, this book provides a repeating circle diagram (see figure 4.1) that allows you to see at once the emerging evidence-based trends of cannabis chemotypes, indicated by the grayscale, recommended for that type of pain. The darker the shade of gray, the more evidence exists.

If you have a mismatch between your preference (checkmark) and evidence-based circular charts, always respect your priority. The reader is reminded that all three cannabis chemotypes positively affect pain by numerous, albeit different, mechanisms, many of which are currently under intense scientific exploration. As such, the correlations of your checkmarks represent only select results we have to date that are subject to change as new data becomes available. Thus your preferred choice may still be beneficial to you.

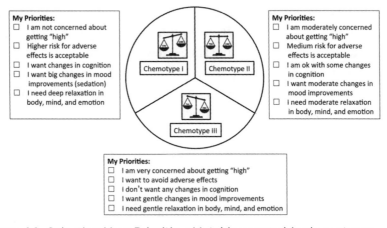

My Priorities:
- ☐ I am not concerned about getting "high"
- ☐ Higher risk for adverse effects is acceptable
- ☐ I want changes in cognition
- ☐ I want big changes in mood improvements (sedation)
- ☐ I need deep relaxation in body, mind, and emotion

My Priorities:
- ☐ I am moderately concerned about getting "high"
- ☐ Medium risk for adverse effects is acceptable
- ☐ I am ok with some changes in cognition
- ☐ I want moderate changes in mood improvements
- ☐ I need moderate relaxation in body, mind, and emotion

My Priorities:
- ☐ I am very concerned about getting "high"
- ☐ I want to avoid adverse effects
- ☐ I don't want any changes in cognition
- ☐ I want gentle changes in mood improvements
- ☐ I need gentle relaxation in body, mind, and emotion

Figure 4.1. Selecting Your Priorities: Matching cannabis chemotypes

Defining Pain

Upon first considering it, defining pain might seem unnecessary—after all, everybody knows what pain is or, more precisely, what it feels like. However, with more thought, it quickly becomes apparent that a more discerning definition of pain and some of the related terms helps us discern not just the location of and reason for the pain, but also the best possible responses to alleviating it. Therefore, it is useful to look at what pain is, what specific types of pains are most common, how pain is processed or blocked, how to find effective analgesia, and, of course, ultimately how to release and heal the pain, if possible.

In general, pain is an unpleasant physical, mental, and emotional experience that is linked to real or maybe even only expected damage to the body or psyche. When we experience pain, what is actually happening can be broken down into pain's common denominators—that is, the separation or loss of something (physical ability, power, love, connection) and a simultaneous desire to have it back.

In mere physical terms, pain is caused by trauma from thermal forces (heat or cold), mechanical forces (pressure, tearing, cutting), chemical forces (acids, bases, toxins), or radiation (UV light, microwaves, or other ionizing radiation such as X-rays).

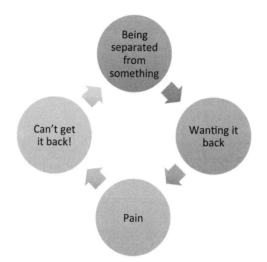

In the most general nonphysical terms, pain requires awareness and consciousness. A paraplegic who has lost sensation below her navel will not feel pain in her feet. Or, as another example, have you ever noticed how pain (physical, mental, and emotional) seems to fade away or diminish when you shift your awareness to watching a movie that is exciting to you? And, of course, everybody knows that pain ends when your consciousness disappears into the deep slumber of sleep or when you become unconscious by means of an anesthetic or a knockout punch. Unfortunately, most of the time as soon as we wake up, so does our pain. While it can be argued that to experience pain we need to be conscious and aware of it, there is more to it.

The experience of pain is uniquely subjective. Virtually no two people will experience pain induced by the same means the same way. That is because we each have a different relationship to pain. We assign meaning, a story, or a narrative to the experience of pain, which directly influences all aspects of pain: intensity, response, duration, and even the length of regeneration of the damage or healing of the trauma causing it. For instance, believing oneself to be in a safe environment can reduce the experience of pain no matter how severe the injury,[197] while simply looking at a painful spot through a magnifying lens will increase swelling and pain.[198] This subjective experience of pain involves a variety of neurochemical mechanisms and different regions of the brain that register the location of pain (somatosensory), compare it to past experiences, determine the urgency of the response and best course of action (cognitive aspects), then signal and execute the response (motivational system) and process the associated emotional material (affective aspects of the brain).

Pain research differentiations and terminologies are voluminous and beyond the scope of this book. As such, some of the specificity and complexity is traded for ease of use and practicality, especially when it comes to making more informed decisions about which analgesic regimen may best suit your needs for effective pain control and safety.

A few basic distinctions are especially relevant. Two terms, *central pain* and *peripheral pain,* refer to the location of the nervous system that is affected. **Central pain** issues are derived from damage (lesions) to the central nervous system (brain and spinal cord). Central pains are typically associated with an underlying pathology such as a spinal cord injury, a stroke, or multiple sclerosis. **Peripheral pain** is associated with damage done to the peripheral nervous system (nerves outside the brain and spinal cord—primarily the limbs). The term **neuropathy** is sometimes added to describe both central and peripheral pains, as in central or peripheral neuropathic pain. It is based on the Latin word *nervus* ("nerve") and the Greek word *pathos* (depending on which dictionary one uses, defined as "calamity," "affliction," or "suffering"). Central and peripheral pains are specifically addressed in more detail later in this chapter.

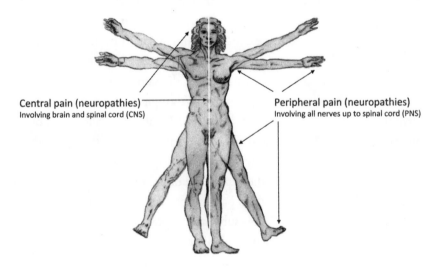

Central pain (neuropathies)
Involving brain and spinal cord (CNS)

Peripheral pain (neuropathies)
Involving all nerves up to spinal cord (PNS)

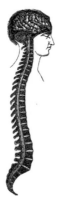

Central Pain and Neuropathies
Selected Scientific Evidence for Effective Pain Control: A Brief Review

Opioids: poor–possible[199]
Cannabinoids: possible[200]

Central pains or neuropathies primarily affect nerves and surrounding areas in the brain and spinal cord, also known as the central nervous system (CNS). There are peripheral neuropathies as well, where the nerve damage occurs in less central areas of the body (see the next section).

In general, opioids don't work very well on chronic central pains,[201] so physicians commonly prescribe anticonvulsant and antidepressant drugs, with varying degrees of analgesic success.[202] A study conducted at the University of California, San Francisco, in 1998 demonstrated that a section of brain-stem circuitry, the rostral ventromedial medulla, found to be contributing to the analgesic effects of opioids, is also involved in cannabinoid-initiated pain-reducing effects. The synthetic cannabinoids used were a potent CB1 antagonist (SR141716A) and a potent both CB1- and CB2-activating agonist (WIN55,212-2). Results showed that analgesia produced by cannabinoids and opioids involves similar brain-stem circuitry, and that cannabinoids are indeed centrally acting analgesics by a mechanism not fully understood.[203] In addition, researchers conducting a review hypothesized that CB2 activation in neuropathologies such as central pain-related conditions may increase the building of new nerve cells (neurogenesis) and as such may play a therapeutic role in central neuropathies.[204]

The neurogenesis hypothesis finds potential support by the findings of a randomized, double-blind, placebo-controlled trial conducted on 66 patients with multiple sclerosis (MS) and central pain who used a chemotype-II (with relatively equal parts THC and CBD) whole-plant cannabis-based oromucosal spray. Each spray delivered 2.7 mg of THC and 2.5 mg of CBD, and patients were instructed to use the spray for pain as needed to a maximum of 48 sprays per 24 hours. Of the 64 patients who completed the trial, 34 actually received the cannabis-based medication. Results showed that "cannabis-based medicine is effective in reducing pain and sleep disturbance in patients with multiple sclerosis–related central neuropathic pain and is mostly well tolerated."[205]

These results were confirmed by another a series of double-blind, randomized, placebo-controlled, single-patient crossover trials performed on a total of 24 patients with central pains (18 with multiple sclerosis, 4 with spinal-cord injury, 1 with brachial plexus damage, and 1 with limb amputation due to neurofibromatosis). Cannabis-based medications were administered also as an oromucosal spray of the chemotype-II variety (with an equal ratio of THC:CBD). Patients were instructed to use as many sprays as needed to achieve analgesia but to stop when unwanted effects occurred. Results showed that pain relief of THC and CBD was significantly superior to placebo.[206]

Brachial plexus root avulsion (a.k.a. brachial plexus lesion) is a central pain-based condition that occurs when a cervical (neck) nerve exiting the spine and extending toward the armpit ruptures, either in part or completely. Perhaps needless to say, it is extremely painful and commonly very resistant to analgesia. A randomized, double-blind, placebo-controlled, three-period crossover study conducted on 48 patients with some form of brachial plexus root avulsion with intractable pain despite analgesic regimens gave participants either placebo, a chemotype-II oromucosal spray (with equal amounts of THC and CBD), or a chemotype-I spray (with THC only). Researchers tested for average pain and quality-of-life improvements. Results showed statistically significant improvements in both pain and quality of sleep.[207]

A crossover, randomized, placebo-controlled human laboratory experiment using vaporized cannabis containing either placebo or 2.9 percent or 6.7 percent THC was conducted on 42 patients with neuropathic pain associated with spinal cord injury or disease. Patients were given 4 puffs and a second dose 3 hours later consisting of totals averaging 4 to 8 puffs. Results showed significant analgesic effects for both the lower and the higher concentration of THC in the vaporized cannabis.[208]

Review Summary: Taken together, the results of the studies noted in the text suggest that each chemotype of cannabis may provide some therapeutic function, albeit by different physiological means. If confirmed in humans, CB2 activation may contribute to neurogenesis, meaning that it could potentially stimulate the growth of new nerve cells. However, the emphasis of the currently available high-quality human trials is on the analgesic efficacy of chemotype I as well as chemotype II for central pains.

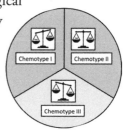

Peripheral Pain and Neuropathies
Selected Scientific Evidence for Effective Pain Control: A Brief Review

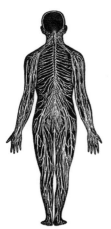

Opioids: poor[209]
Cannabinoids: possible–good[210]

Peripheral pain or peripheral neuropathy refers primarily to pain in more outlying locations of the body leading up to the spinal cord and brain. Peripheral neuropathies are generally produced by an underlying disease or condition such as diabetes or HIV/AIDS, nutritional deficiency such as lack of vitamin B12, certain microbial infections such as *Herpes zoster* and leprosy, and chronic degenerative conditions that include autoimmune diseases, vasculitis, and cancer; or the pains arise as common adverse effects of numerous pharmaceutical drugs (Cisplatin, Dilantin, Cipro). These pains tend to be chronic in nature. Here, even though opioids may be effective in cases or episodes of acute peripheral pain, in chronic cases opioids tend to have limited effectiveness. One retrospective population-based cohort study discovered that outcomes were worse for patients with neuropathic pain who received long-term opioid treatment compared to those receiving short-term opioid treatment.[211] A recent systematic review and meta-analysis arrived at the conclusion that the evidence for opioid use for neuropathic pains is weak, and strong opioids were recommended only as a third-line option after other options were exhausted first.[212] Another study considering the risk versus benefits of opioids in the treatment of neuropathies found that "long-term opioid therapy did not improve functional status but rather was associated with a higher risk of subsequent opioid dependency and overdose."[213]

In contrast, numerous studies indicate a positive therapeutic potential of various cannabinoid preparations in neuropathies in general[214] and in cases of diabetic neuropathies[215] and AIDS-related neuropathies in particular.[216] Another condition that may benefit from the analgesic qualities of cannabis in a treatment regime is allodynia,[217] a type of neuropathic pain associated with painful sensations that normally would not cause pain, such as gentle touch, movement, or a feeling of warmth. Patients suffering from allodynia experience hurt or burning pains instead of the usual feeling. This type of pain is usually associated with an underlying condition such as zoster, fibromyalgia, or migraine.

A double-blind, placebo-controlled trial conducted by a group of researchers at the University of California, Davis, Medical Center examined the effects of low- and "medium"-dose cannabis administration in the treatment of neuropathic pains. A total of 0.8 g (800 mg) of cannabis was placed in a Volcano vaporizer, vaporized, and collected in the vape bag. For this experiment, researchers instructed the patients to inhale for 5 seconds, hold for 10 seconds, exhale, and wait for 40 seconds before repeating the inhalation procedure to a total of 4 inhalations. Three hours later, patients repeated the procedure but had the option to inhale up to 8 times. The low dose of cannabis contained ~1.3% THC and the "medium" dose contained ~3.5% THC (no information was given regarding CBD content). Results indicated that vaporized cannabis, even at low doses, may produce effective analgesia for patients with treatment-resistant neuropathic pains.[218]

A review of fifteen double-blind, placebo-controlled trials conducted on human patients suffering from chronic neuropathic pains (a total of 1,619 patients) concluded that cannabinoids were superior to placebo in the reduction of neuropathic pains. Ten of the studies used a plant-derived oromucosal spray with equal amounts of THC and CBD (chemotype II), three studies employed the synthetic cannabinoids nabilone and dronabinol (with THC only, thus chemotype I), and two studies used cannabis flower.[219] The chemotypes tested to date in the context of treating chronic neuropathic pains in human trials included primarily chemotypes II and to a lesser degree chemotype I.

Review Summary: Taken together, the results of the human trials suggest that the chemotypes tested to date in the context of treating chronic neuropathic pains included primarily chemotype II and to a lesser degree chemotype I.

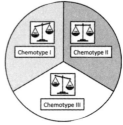

Treating Acute versus Chronic Pain

Acute pain and **chronic pain** describe the immediate nature of the pain, and the terms are mostly self-explanatory. The word *acute* is derived from the Latin *acutus,* meaning "sharp," and is used to describe an intense or urgent type of pain. The word *chronic* has its origin in the Greek *khronos,* meaning "time." Chronic pain is usually considered to last more than twelve weeks and is generally less intense than acute pain. Both central and peripheral pains can be acute or chronic in nature, and this aspect often determines the best approach to medication.

In cases of acute injuries (especially to the periphery), after surgeries, or with advanced end-of-life cancer-based pains, opioids commonly provide useful analgesia.[220] In contrast, there is little evidence to date that using cannabinoid-based medication in cases of acute pain is very helpful.[221] Nor would many (if any) anecdotes from millions of people's personal experience attest to the great usefulness of cannabis in such a situation.

Bottom line: opium-based medicines are your go-to option for this, no question. The type of pain relief suggested in this book is for chronic pain, which persists over time but not at the emergency or intolerable levels of acute pain. Chronic pain can include mental and emotional states such as distress, depression, and hopelessness, among others. Treatment of chronic pain must involve lower doses of opioids than those used for acute pain; otherwise addiction, resistance, and withdrawal may result. This is why cannabis can help in the treatment of chronic pain—it complements and augments the effects of opioids, allowing for lower dosages, and it supplies additional benefits of endocannabinoids. Ideally, using cannabis as a pain-relief adjunct or major element of one's program is part of a holistic approach that includes examining mind-body connections, making healthy lifestyle changes, participating in counseling or therapy, and many other possibilities for deeper and more complete healing of the roots of physical, mental, and emotional pain.

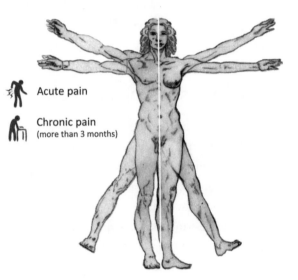

Acute pain

Chronic pain
(more than 3 months)

Acute Pain

Selected Scientific Evidence for Effective Pain Control: A Brief Review

Opioids: good[222]
Cannabinoids: poor to possible[223]

While cannabis is generally acknowledged as more useful for chronic than acute pain, research is ongoing. One study suggested that CBD might reduce incision type pains in rodents,[224] while another animal experiment demonstrated that CBD may enhance the analgesic effects of THC.[225] A trial conducted on human patients undergoing dental extractions suggested that intravenously (IV) administered THC (0.022 mg/kg and 0.044 mg/kg) produced inconsistent and relatively poor analgesic results in acute settings.[226]

Review Summary: No high-quality studies to date indicate the success of using cannabis in different forms, cannabinoid ratios, concentrations, or other routes of administration in the treatment of acute pain.

Chronic Pain

Selected Scientific Evidence for Effective Pain Control: A Brief Review

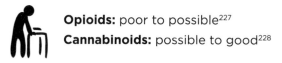

Opioids: poor to possible[227]
Cannabinoids: possible to good[228]

Evidence shows that opioids do not work very well on chronic pains.[229] In contrast, accumulating evidence suggests that patients suffering from certain chronic pains may achieve significant relief from the therapeutic use of cannabinoids.

For instance, a randomized, double-blind, placebo-controlled crossover trial conducted on 34 patients with chronic (mostly neuropathic) pain for a period of twelve weeks demonstrated that metered sprays containing THC (2.5 mg per spray) and containing THC and CBD (2.5 mg THC plus 2.5 mg CBD per spray) were effective in relieving chronic pains. Patients were instructed to self-medicate as needed. Researchers and patients acknowledged a brief learning curve to achieve effective symptom relief while avoiding adverse effects. The effective spray usage averaged roughly 8 sprays per day for THC only (total of 20 mg) and about 7 sprays for combined THC and CBD (17.5 mg THC and 17.5 mg CBD). Patients were able to medicate in public without attracting unwelcome attention from others. Researchers reported that side effects were not substantially different from those seen with most other psychoactive drugs used in pain management.[230]

As another example, a randomized, placebo-controlled, double-blind crossover trial conducted on 21 patients with chronic neuropathic pains (some with hyperalgesia and others with allodynia) utilized ajulemic acid (CT-3), a synthetic analog of a metabolite of delta-9-THC. Like THC, ajulemic acid binds to CB1 (with high affinity, ~4 times stronger than THC) and CB2 receptor sites (with moderate affinity, ~half the strength of THC).[231] Results showed that ajulemic acid was able to produce analgesic effects without the occurrence of major adverse effects.[232]

Let's briefly consider the evidence of the largest trial to date, a risk versus benefit analysis conducted over the course of one year on 431 patients with chronic nonmalignant pain. Participants were roughly divided into two groups, one using cannabis and the other not. Researchers examined the effectiveness and safety of cannabis with a focus on mild, moderate, and serious adverse effects, and they also monitored secondary safety measurements on lung and neurocognitive function, standard hematology, biochemistry, and renal, liver, and endocrine function. Results showed that a standardized dose of dried cannabis flowers (12.5% THC; no CBD values given) up to a relatively high dose of an average of 2.5 g per day (with a recommended top limit of 5 g per day) for a year produced a significant reduction in pain intensity among the cannabis users over the control group. Cannabis appears in this study to have a reasonable safety profile with an increased risk of temporary mild to moderate adverse effects (such as altered state of consciousness, forgetfulness, cough, euphoria, dizziness, and nausea) in the cannabis group.[233]

Review Summary: Taken together, these study results suggest that observed analgesic effects in cases of chronic (neuropathic) pains were most likely modulated by THC, or by products containing both THC and CBD in a relatively equal ratio. Ingested THC was used in 2.5 mg increments to a maximum of 20 mg per day. Inhaled cannabis flower was inhaled as needed to a maximum of 2.5 g (containing 12.5% THC, which is a little more than 300 mg THC). Similar results were observed for ingestion of THC and CBD at equal ratios of increments of 2.5 mg each of THC and CBD to a maximum of 17.5 mg.

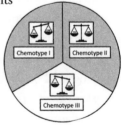

Taking the variables of absorption into account, research suggests a ratio (ingestion:inhalation) of about 1:6.[234] That is, for every 1 mg of ingested THC, about 6 mg of inhaled THC may be necessary to achieve a similar effect. Please keep in mind that this ratio is an estimate, to be considered with appropriate caution. It was derived mathematically from averages of different study results, each with ranges that had large margins. The takeaway? Use much less when ingesting.

Remember, the ranges are based on limited available scientific literature to date. In fact, a number of preclinical studies suggest that CBD may reduce chronic pain if underlying inflammatory conditions are part of the chronic pain picture.[235]

Additional Useful Distinctions of Pain and the Evidence for Treating Them

Along with acute versus chronic and central versus peripheral pains, another three terms suggest underlying mechanisms responsible for causing the pain: **nociceptive, inflammatory,** and **pathological pains.**[236] You may want to think of a traffic-light analogy. A red light is nociceptive pain that demands you "stop"—it gets your immediate attention. Inflammatory pain is the yellow light giving you a warning, and where a green light would normally be, you get a broken light that flickers at best with ongoing pathological pain.

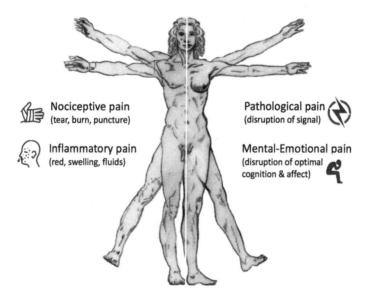

Nociceptive pain
(tear, burn, puncture)

Inflammatory pain
(red, swelling, fluids)

Pathological pain
(disruption of signal)

Mental-Emotional pain
(disruption of optimal
cognition & affect)

Nociceptive Pain
Selected Scientific Evidence for Effective Pain Control: A Brief Review

 Opioids: good in acute self-limiting injuries,[237] poor–possible in chronic conditions[238]
Cannabinoids: possible[239]

Nociceptive pain is caused by a noxious stimulus such as a burn. More specifically, nociceptive pain is produced when long sensory nerve fibers (axons) pick up a painful stimulus such as excess heat from the body's periphery. A nociceptor is a type of receptor located at the ends of these sensory axons that responds to potentially damaging stimuli, and the process of perceiving and feeling this pain when a nociceptor is stimulated is called nociception. Physiologically, it is composed of four processes: transduction, transmission, modulation, and perception. It is in the modulation that medicine plays its role.

The noxious stimulus travels from the site of origin along the full length of the axon, which can be up to three feet long, until it is transduced up the spinal cord and farther to the brain's pain-processing center. Here the brain interprets the signal. The brain determines that the pain is significant and sends a message all the way down another axon pathway to the corresponding muscles. The leg pulls up the foot that was touching the fire. All this happens near instantaneously. For the pain of a burn injury like this, opioids tend to work well, especially if the pain is acute (intense) and the drugs are used for a limited time.[240] Acute nociceptive pain tends to be short in duration, and once the causative agent is removed and the body is allowed to repair itself without another complication, healing will take its course.

However, if nociceptive pain has a maintaining cause such as in patients with osteoarthritis (OA) or rheumatoid arthritis (RA), the efficacy of opioid use is subject to debate, and a careful risk versus benefit analysis of the patient's experience and the opinion of the treating physician should be carried out. Regarding analgesic efficacy of opioids in cases of OA, a review of 20 randomized placebo-controlled studies discovered that the actual average reduction in pain intensity was small.[241]

In contrast, evidence is beginning to suggest that endocannabinoid engagement via a variety of receptor mechanisms can positively influence nociception in patient populations suffering from these underlying conditions. For instance, a randomized, double-blind, placebo-controlled crossover trial investigated the effects of a chemotype-II oromucosal spray (containing equal amounts of THC and CBD) on a group of 17 patients suffering from MS-based nociceptive pain. Results provided evidence that cannabinoids positively modulated the nociceptive system in these patients.[242]

Research conducted on 32 patients with OA and 13 more suffering from RA suggested that CB1 and CB2 receptor sites as well as endocannabinoids such as anandamide are abundantly found in patients' affected tissues and as such are posited to be a novel target for the treatment of noxious pain associated with these conditions.[243]

A review provides new evidence that cannabinoids hitherto believed to generate antinociceptive effects mainly via activation of CB1 receptor sites[244] are part of an emerging and more complex mechanism involving CB1 modulation of neurotransmitters such as serotonin and norepinephrine to produce antinociceptive effects.[245]

Review Summary: Taken together, these results suggest cannabis chemotypes ranging between I and II.

Chemotype I — *Chemotype II* — *Chemotype III*

Inflammatory Pain

Selected Scientific Evidence for Effective Pain Control: A Brief Review

Opioids: poor–possible[246]
Cannabinoids: good[247]

Inflammation is a natural and necessary response of the healing process. In fact, without an inflammatory response, injuries would not heal. **Inflammatory pain** is caused by tissue swelling, the function of which is to activate and facilitate movement of immune cells to the affected tissue until it is repaired. This involves swelling, heat, redness, pain, and the impairment of function at the affected site—all reminders to nurse the spot until the healing process is complete.

Inflammation can be acute or chronic. Acute inflammation tends to be time-limited and ends when the damaged tissue is healed. On the other hand, chronic inflammation may produce varied responses and be more of a long-term issue, especially if there is a maintaining cause, such as the presence of a foreign object; when an invading organism or toxin cannot be expelled or continuously reappears; when an injury is not allowed to heal and instead is constantly agitated; or when an overreactive immune system attacks itself, such as in rheumatoid arthritis.

While the use of topical opioids in the treatment of certain peripheral inflammatory conditions has demonstrated some therapeutic potential,[248] evidence shows that opioids can cause pain sensation to increase by releasing pro-inflammatory cytokines.[249] As such, the evidence for the systemic use of opioids for inflammatory pain and inflammatory-based conditions is limited and subject to debate. Additionally, research suggests that nonsteroidal anti-inflammatory drugs (NSAIDs) are a safer alternative to the use of opioids in the treatment of inflammatory-based pains.[250] Chronic use of NSAIDs has its own significant set of problems, so it's saying a lot when those are safer than opioids.

CB2 receptor sites are abundantly present in cells of the immune system and are intricately involved in modulating a variety of immune-related responses, including inflammation-based pains.[251] Mounting evidence also implicates a number of other endocannabinoid-based components, such as ionotropic cannabinoid receptors (TRPs), neurotransmitter modulation such as opioid receptors, peroxisome proliferator-activated receptors (PPARs), and anandamide and the associated hydrolyzing enzyme FAAH in producing anti-inflammatory actions.[252]

Significant evidence shows that cannabinoid-based therapies can improve inflammatory-based pain.[253] To date, the scientific evidence supports the position that cannabis constituents are immune-modulating agents, affecting a variety of immune cells by a number of different mechanisms, and as such produce in general a reduction in pro-inflammatory cytokines and an increase in anti-inflammatory cytokines. This dual action is of significance, as some conditions are caused by an overactive immune system while others are initiated by an underactive immune response. For instance, an immune system that is turning on itself underlies cases of rheumatoid arthritis, type 1 diabetes, and systemic sclerosis.[254]

Research discovered that engaging the endocannabinoid system may provide a novel mechanism to therapeutically influence chronic inflammatory-based conditions such as arthritis,[255] atherosclerosis,[256] interstitial cystitis,[257] rheumatoid arthritis,[258] gastro-esophageal reflux disease (GERD),[259] inflammatory bowel disease (IBD, IBS, and colitis),[260] pancreatitis,[261] and periodontitis.[262]

Review Summary: Given the vast variety of conditions that share inflammatory pains, and given the number of mechanisms and means by which cannabinoids up- or down-regulate immune responses accordingly, specific chemotype-based suggestions must be done on a case-by-case basis, which is beyond the scope of this book. As such, a broad evidence-based recommendation for inflammation-based pains, presented in this review, ranges from a chemotype I to a chemotype III. This implies that almost every type of cannabis can help inflammation to some degree.

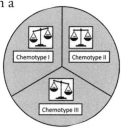

Pathological Pain
Selected Scientific Evidence for Effective Pain Control: A Brief Review

Opioids: poor[263]
Cannabinoids: possible–good[264]

The Greek words *pathos* ("suffering") and *logia* ("the study of") build the term **pathological pain.** This type of pain is characterized by an interruption of the pain-signaling process or pathway. When the normal pathways are dysfunctional, pathological pain results. This type of pain is commonly associated with a very low pain threshold, responds poorly to orthodox treatments, and is thought to result primarily from amplified central nerve signaling.[265] Pathological pains are associated with conditions that are able to produce abnormal pain signaling, such as diabetes, multiple sclerosis, and amyotrophic lateral sclerosis (ALS).

Glial cells have been discovered to be significantly involved in the development of pathological pains.[266] These are nervous-system supportive cells, comprising astrocytes, oligodendrocytes, ependymal, and microglia cells. Glial cells form myelin, the protective sheathing surrounding nerve cells, and support, protect, and work toward homeostasis (balance).

An experiment conducted on rodents demonstrated that opioids tend to work poorly on pathological pains, while in contrast, the cannabis-based constituent THC has been shown to be a superior option for alleviating pathological pains.[267] While this has not been fully studied in humans, researchers have noted that activation of CB1 receptor sites reduces pathological pain but also produces a high effect or changes in cognition considered by some an adverse effect.[268] To address these concerns, an experiment conducted at Indiana University explored a novel CB1 positive allosteric modulator (called GAT211) in the context of pathological pains. Results indicated a potentially novel agent able to alleviate pathological pains without affecting the state of consciousness.[269]

Review Summary: Given the present evidence, and in the absence of more trials examining the efficacy of cannabinoid-based medications, one can tentatively conclude that a chemotype-I based product would be most effective for pathological pains.

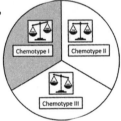

The All-Too-Often Forgotten Faces of Pain: Mental-Emotional Suffering

Your pain is the breaking of the shell that encloses your understanding.

—KHALIL GIBRAN

In working up to addressing addictions, vulnerabilities to addictions, the limitations of the current models of addictions, and how to realize a new and more complex approach to breaking the cycle of addictions—as well as how to significantly increase chances of preventing them in the first place—it becomes important to explore the all-too-often forgotten aspects of pain. I am referring to pain that is not primarily physical.

Mental-Emotional Pain
Selected Scientific Evidence for Effective Pain Control in Cases: A Brief Review

 Opioids: Makes you forget about it temporarily but does not change the cause.
Cannabinoids: Can set stage for exploration and revelation. Can make intolerable emotion OK. May assist in resolution.

Similarly to physical pain, mental and emotional pain are basic and very subjective human experiences. And while everybody has this form of pain from time to time (and sometimes for long times), defining it is even more difficult than accurately defining physical pain. This difficulty is reflected in the approach of orthodox medicine. The American Psychiatric Association has compiled a list of mental and emotional disorders in its regularly updated *Diagnostic and Statistical Manual of Mental Disorders (DSM-5),* but the APA and DSM do not define mental or emotional pain. In fact, the word *pain* only shows up a few times throughout its voluminous pages. Earlier editions employed the term *Pain Disorders,* now in the latest edition renamed *Somatic Symptoms and Related Disorders.* The closest the *DSM-5* comes to defining mental-emotional pain is when it explores some of the dimensions of grief, bereavement, and post–traumatic stress disorder.

For instance, grief is considered normal as long it lasts only for days and not weeks. But what if it lasts longer? According to the latest *DSM-5,* a person grieving longer than two weeks is considered to have a pharmacologically treatable mental disorder called a major depressive disorder.[270] But is an antidepressive pill going to cure grief that lasts longer than a couple of weeks?

A bereaved person experiences the loss of a loved one, for example. The simultaneous separation and longing for their return causes mental and emotional pain. The stronger the longing, the stronger the pain. Symptoms may include: insomnia, depression, anger, anxiety, or lack of appetite. When the mental-emotional process of grief is allowed its due time, when the inevitable changes are processed, integrated, and eventually accepted, grief will find its natural end—ideally leaving us with a beautiful sadness along with peaceful acceptance of what is. However, sometime people don't complete their pain process. Sometimes people get stuck in one phase or another. What is going to happen to that pain of separation, that pain of devastating loss, or that pain of intense loneliness? The tendency of many people is the same tendency now proposed by the *DSM:* medicate. Why is that?

Earlier in this chapter we described the basic steps of how pain is processed. In this oversimplified example, the brain registers pain (being separated from something and wanting it back), compares it to past experiences, and determines the urgency of the response and best course of action. When comparing, the brain remembers that taking a pain pill helped. The brain issues a directive to seek the pill, take the pill, and expect relief, which brings us to opioids and cannabinoids.

In ancient Greece, opium was called "the destroyer of grief." In Homer's epic poem *The Odyssey,* opium is described as follows:

> Helen, meanwhile, the child of Zeus, had a happy thought. Into the bowl in which their wine was mixed, she slipped a drug that had the power of robbing grief and anger of their sting and banishing all painful memories. No one that swallowed this dissolved in wine could shed a single tear that day, even for the death of his mother and father, or if they put his brother or his own son to the sword and he were there to see it done.[271]

Opium use, no matter what form, whether as morphine, fentanyl, or heroin, replaces not just certain physical pains but also mental-emotional pains such as sorrow, grief, loneliness, guilt, and shame with varying expressions of a "subtle" euphoria. This is especially true when compared to the rambunctious euphoria of alcohol, the giddy euphoria of laughing gas (nitrous oxide), or the hyperstimulated euphoria of methamphetamines, for example.

A review of historical autobiographical firsthand experiences with opium finds descriptions such as the following: consolation of warmth and calmness;

sensations of ease and comfort; the soft, quiet place between wakefulness and sleep; a slow, long-lasting, low-intensity orgasm; or a soft sleep and the end of pain. Obviously, using an opioid medication for a short period, as a treatment for specific acute pains, or for the treatments of end-of-life patients can be a godsend. But opioid use may extract a significant price.

Common adverse effects can turn chronic, and increasing tolerance may requires larger amounts, thus producing a vulnerability to developing addiction, along with the very real risk of a fatal overdose. And, similarly to being stuck in a phase of pain or grief, the opium-based drug does not resolve grief permanently as does a natural conclusion that tends to appear somewhere during the journey through pain. The natural process of pain and grief usually comes to a place of transcendence that sets us free from the worst of the pain or grief while also changing us, hopefully for the better.

Clinical observations reveal that opioid-dependent individuals, in addition to experiencing physical pain, commonly suffer from painful emotions that reinforce the use of drugs to self-medicate.[272] Thus addressing pain, not just in its physical form but also in terms of affect (emotional aspects) and cognition (mental aspects), can combine to create a more complete pathway or map to ending addiction. Unfortunately, a medical system accustomed to managing pain with drugs often considers emotions as getting in the way. But what if emotions are the way, or at least part of the way? What if, instead of medicating them into temporary oblivion, we listen, learn, understand, and integrate the changes residing in the heart of pain?

While opioids can induce temporary relief from mental-emotional pain, they do not resolve it, nor do they constructively change the narrative of pain. And while we all need a Band-Aid from time to time, while we all need to escape or manage pain in some situations, as soon as the opioid wears off, affectual pain often returns with all its devastating force.

In contrast, working with cannabis can help mitigate these symptoms and assist in resolving them. Take, for example, the emerging evidence that patients suffering from certain symptoms commonly found in grief such as insomnia, depression, anger, anxiety, or lack of appetite are switching more and more from pharmaceuticals to cannabis.[273] A great number of cannabis-using patients find relief for insomnia,[274] depression,[275] anger,[276] or the lack of appetite,[277] and it would appear that the scientific evidence supports and validates their experiences.

Review Summary: Each of the studies reviewed in this section uses one of the three cannabis chemotypes to test a variety of therapeutic effects manifested by a great variety of mechanisms unique to each chemotype.

All three chemotypes may show promise, depending on your individual situation. Use your preference for what kind of cannabis experience you wish to have as a starting point and keep some notes to provide a way to monitor what it was like and what you learned to fine-tune your future direction and choices.

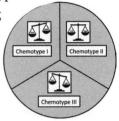

The Example of PTSD

Let's first look at another example of mental-emotional pain: that of post–traumatic stress disorder (PTSD). The orthodox medical system classifies PTSD as a mental disorder that measurably and negatively affects body, mind, and emotions.[278] It is associated with sudden trauma or trauma that was repeated over long periods of time. People vulnerable to developing PTSD include those who had a direct experience or even just witnessed an extreme traumatic event such as acts of war, police brutalities, famine, earthquake, tsunami, assault, abuse, rape, kidnapping, torture, plane crash, explosions, life-threatening illness, or any situation involving the threat of death, extreme fear, dread, and helplessness.

In World War I it was known as "shell shock"; in World War II it was termed "battle fatigue"; and the modern name, PTSD, was coined during the years of the Vietnam War when thousands of soldiers came home suffering from a collection of common chronic symptoms manifesting in body (insomnia, tension, headaches), mind (flashbacks, nightmares, lost capacity to trust, paranoia, irritability, inability to concentrate, negative beliefs about self, hurtful self-talk), and emotions (guilt, depression, shame, fear, numbness, inability to be close to loved ones). It was not until 1980 that PTSD was defined, codified, and included in the *Diagnostic and Statistical Manual of Mental Disorders*.

Of course, people exposed to the same traumatic event tend to respond differently. Due to the range of personal resilience and the variety of chosen narrative we assign to the event, some may experience only mild and passing symptoms, while others may progress to developing full-blown PTSD. And while certainly not everybody with PTSD reaches for drugs to self-medicate their most stressful symptoms, evidence shows that a great number of people who are addicted to opioids also suffer from PTSD.[279] Here is what's instructive: when addicted patients with PTSD were taught to identify and cope with emotions and thoughts sourced in pain, it produced a clear reduction of substance use.[280] In direct contrast, there were no such improvements in symptoms of PTSD when physical addiction symptoms were treated first. These findings indicate the importance of addressing the cognitive and emotional aspects of pain.[281]

While not every person with PTSD has a history of acute or chronic physical pain, a great number of them do. However, and perhaps most importantly, what most patients dealing with acute or chronic pains have in common with patients suffering from PTSD are expressions of mental and emotional anguish and an increased vulnerability to developing addiction.

By definition and in theory, trauma, pain, PTSD, and opioid addictions are distinct terms that have unique physical, mental, and emotional characteristics. In reality, however, all are often closely linked.[282] For instance, hypervigilance in PTSD may look like opioid withdrawal symptoms. Consider this partial list of other common and overlapping or converging symptoms of opioid addiction and PTSD: physical symptoms (fitful sleep with sweating, insomnia, overly sensitive to sensory stimulation, reduced appetite, increased heart rate and blood pressure); mental symptoms (hyper-alertness, irritability, inexplicable fear, anxiety, lack of focus, lost memories, passivity); and emotional symptoms (guilt, worthlessness, shame, numbness, intense anger with little or no provocation).

As such, the evidence suggests a dynamic relationship, especially between PTSD and addiction.[283] Researchers posit that this relationship is based on shared neurobiological circuitry and pathophysiological mechanisms.[284] You may ask why this is important. Its significance lies in the clinical observations that addressing them together in a therapeutic and integrated fashion is most likely to produce the best results in getting well and staying well.[285] It is also significant because, as you will see, engaging the endocannabinoid system in a therapeutic fashion can constructively support this process in all of its complexities.

The Role of Beliefs in Mental-Emotional Pain

Grief and the ongoing struggles of PTSD are clear examples of mental-emotional pain. Other forms of pain are not so obvious to others. A young woman loses her first love and longs to hold her again. An author inadvertently pushes the wrong button on his computer and loses his entire manuscript; he feels a part of him has died with it. And what about the mental-emotional pain that is associated with a physically traumatic event and physical pain, such as that of the torn Achilles tendon that forces the soccer player to give up his identity as a star athlete in his prime? Or the shock, pain, and separation from who we have been that is often referred to as midlife crisis? Also, consider opioid-induced hyperalgesia (hyperkatifeia): the hypothesis that the analgesic misuse (too much or for too long) produces a hypersensitivity to mental-emotional pain, which in turn intensifies the experience of physical pain.[286] The latter is not to be confused with allodynia, a painful experience of a sensation that normally would not hurt, which is a condition that also benefits from endocannabinoid-based neuromodulation[287] (see "Nociceptive Pain" in chapter 4).

While some of us are resilient and recover quickly, others may be devastated by tragic life events, and it may take years to heal. The difference, at least in part, may be found in our subjective narrative of pain that is largely responsible for how we process, integrate, and learn from a painful experience. Let's take the processing of beliefs, for example. Beliefs aren't right or wrong, but they can have measurable biological consequences that are especially relevant for healing chronic pain and addiction.

Beliefs that induce guilt, harbored anger, insistence on punishment for perceived wrongs, hopelessness, prejudice, or bias, for example, tend to chronically increase sympathetic nervous system reactions such as fight, flight, or freeze responses. In chronic stress states we are constantly exposed to stress hormones such as cortisol (stress), glutamate (excitation), or epinephrine (fear) that not only increase heart rate and blood pressure but inhibit our natural capacity to reduce inflammation, due to an increase in pro-inflammatory cytokines; diminish the resilience of our immune system to ward off fungi, bacteria, and viruses; and reduce the presence of endogenous opioids. Each factor alone and certainly in combination may contribute to maintaining and even increasing pain sensations, and this includes opioid withdrawal symptoms.[288]

If, on the other hand, we have or develop beliefs that focus on discernment, curiosity, tempered positivity, hope, forgiveness, gratitude, and compassion, for example, we increase parasympathetic activity called the relaxation response, which is in direct opposition to fight, flight, or freeze, and as such reduces heart rate, blood pressure, and stress hormones. Instead of being drenched in stress hormones, the body will actually increase levels of serotonin (happy, feeling good), anandamide (ease, bliss), anti-inflammatory cytokines, oxytocin (trust, empathy), endogenous opioids (painkillers), or GABA (relaxation), for example.[289] Each of these changes alone and in combination may contribute to reducing pain intensity and duration as well as opioid withdrawal symptoms.

Here is what is fascinating: Any and all of the communication molecules mentioned are partly or significantly modulated by the endocannabinoid system. Additional good news is that our pain narrative, including the beliefs we hold, are subject to conscious intervention, and producing changes here will support our healing from pain in all spheres of body, mind, and emotion. In other words, consciously identifying unhealthy beliefs and replacing them with healthier ones goes a long way toward enhancing the body's own capcity for healing.

For instance, numerous mindfulness techniques (yoga, breath-focused practices), meditation practices (tai chi, qi gong), spiritual practices (repetitive prayer), or next-generation psychological therapies for chronic pains (cognitive-behavioral treatment)[290] may be used toward developing a healthier and supportive belief system that in turn can support an internal environment that increases our stress resilience in general and reduces pain and opioid withdrawal symptoms specifically. The remaining chapters continue to explore the role of the mind and emotions in healing from pain and vice versa—and the endocannabinoid system's multifaceted role in all these processes. Any effective and complete healing will ultimately have to include both mind and body.

To summarize all this information in a more practical fashion, consider using the following worksheet. It combines relevant evidence-based data and your priorities. Simply fill in all the checkmarks that apply to you and notice if and where your priorities, concerns, and needs concentrate or cluster. More marks collecting beneath one particular cannabis chemotype may be an indication of a likely good starting point for making a more informed decision about what chemotype of cannabis may be best suited for your condition and disposition.

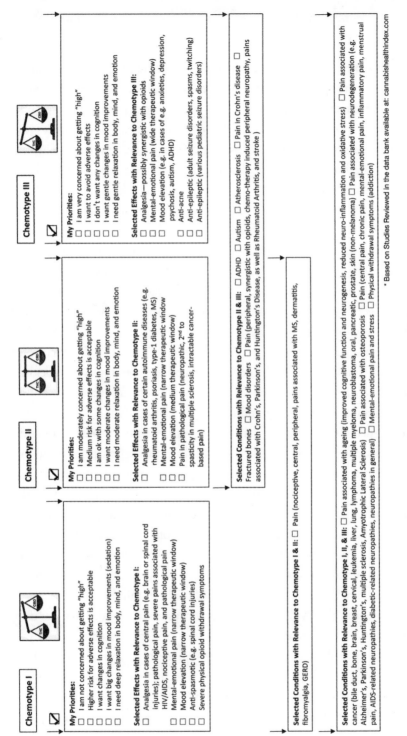

Chemotype I

My Priorities:
- ☐ I am not concerned about getting "high"
- ☐ Higher risk for adverse effects is acceptable
- ☐ I want changes in cognition
- ☐ I want big changes in mood improvements (sedation)
- ☐ I need deep relaxation in body, mind, and emotion

Selected Effects with Relevance to Chemotype I:
- ☐ Analgesia in cases of central pain (e.g. brain or spinal cord injuries); pathological pain, severe pains associated with HIV/AIDS, nociceptive pain, and pathological pain
- ☐ Mental-emotional pain (narrow therapeutic window)
- ☐ Mood elevation (narrow therapeutic window)
- ☐ Anti-spasmotic (e.g. spinal cord injuries)
- ☐ Severe physical opioid withdrawal symptoms

Chemotype II

My Priorities:
- ☐ I am moderately concerned about getting "high"
- ☐ Medium risk for adverse effects is acceptable
- ☐ I am ok with some changes in cognition
- ☐ I want moderate changes in mood improvements
- ☐ I need moderate relaxation in body, mind, and emotion

Selected Effects with Relevance to Chemotype II:
- ☐ Analgesia in cases of certain autoimmune diseases (e.g. rheumatoid arthritis, psoriasis, type-1 diabetes, MS)
- ☐ Mental-emotional pain (narrow therapeutic window
- ☐ Mood elevation (medium therapeutic window)
- ☐ Pain in pathological pain (neuropathic, 2nd to spasticity in multiple sclerosis, intractable cancer-based pain)

Chemotype III

My Priorities:
- ☐ I am very concerned about getting "high"
- ☐ I want to avoid adverse effects
- ☐ I don't want any changes in cognition
- ☐ I want gentle changes in mood improvements
- ☐ I need gentle relaxation in body, mind, and emotion

Selected Effects with Relevance to Chemotype III:
- ☐ Analgesia—possibly synergistic with opioids
- ☐ Mental-emotional pain (wide therapeutic window)
- ☐ Mood elevation (e.g. in cases of e.g. anxieties, depression, psychosis, autism, ADHD)
- ☐ Anti-acne
- ☐ Anti-epileptic (adult seizure disorders, spasms, twitching)
- ☐ Anti-epileptic (various pediatric seizure disorders)

Selected Conditions with Relevance to Chemotype II & III: ☐ ADHD ☐ Autism ☐ Atherosclerosis ☐ Pain in Crohn's disease ☐ Mood disorders ☐ Pain (peripheral, synergistic with opioids, chemo-therapy induced peripheral neuropathy, pains associated with Crohn's, Parkinson's, and Huntington's Disease, as well as Rheumatoid Arthritis, and stroke)

Selected Conditions with Relevance to Chemotype I & II: ☐ Pain (nociceptive, central, peripheral, pains associated with MS, dermatitis, fibromyalgia, GERD)

Selected Conditions with Relevance to Chemotype I, II, & III: ☐ Pain associated with ageing (improved cognitive function and neurogenesis, reduced neuro-inflammation and oxidative stress) ☐ Pain associated with cancer (bile duct, bone, brain, breast, cervical, leukemia, liver, lung, lymphoma, multiple myeloma, neuroblastoma, oral, pancreatic, prostate, skin (non-melanoma) ☐ Pain associated with neurodegeneration (e.g. Alzheimer's, Parkinson's, Huntington's, multiple sclerosis, Amyotrophic Lateral Sclerosis) ☐ Pain (central pain, chronic pain, mental-emotional pain, inflammatory pain, menstrual pain, AIDS-related neuropathies, diabetic-related neuropathies, neuropathies in general) ☐ Mental-emotional pain and stress ☐ Physical withdrawal symptoms (addiction)

* Based on Studies Reviewed in the data bank available at: cannabishealthindex.com

Select Chemotype-Based Effects Relevant to Pain and Opioid Withdrawal

COMMON AND COMPARATIVE EFFECTS AND ADVERSE EFFECTS OF OPIOIDS AND CANNABINOIDS

PHARMACEUTICAL DRUG	EFFECTS AND ADVERSE EFFECTS	OPIOID	CANNABIS

Opium-based analgesics are prescribed for acute and chronic pain. Names include:
 	
  Vicodin
  OxyContin
  oxycodone
  hydrocodone
  fentanyl
  carfentanil
  codeine
  Demerol
  Percodan
  morphine
  heroin is the street version of morphine with about twice its strength.
 	
Opium-based drugs for opioid withdrawal symptoms:
  methadone
 	
Cannabinoid-based pharmaceutical drugs include:
  chemotype I
  dronabinol
  chemotype II
  Sativex
  chemotype III
  Epidiolex
	Common Effects and Adverse Effects		

	analgesia	yes	yes
	relaxation	yes	yes
	euphoria	yes	yes
	"high"	yes	yes
	(may be similar among opium, morphine, heroin, and different between other pharma-based opioids such as methadone or carfentanil, and experience depends on form, route, concentration, and constitution of user)	The opium high is often described as orgasmic but longer-lasting, giving way to pleasure, sedation, relaxation, analgesia, a sleepy dreamlike state void of any pain, fear, worry, or stress.	Appreciation of beauty, art, music, deep thoughts, the "otherworldly," enhanced memory or loss of short-term memory, increase in sensual intensity, visual or auditory shifts of perceptions, mirth, playfulness, more intense food taste, mild psyche-delic effects
	dysphoria (e.g. anxiety, depression)	yes	yes (if dose is too high, may feel anxiety, panic attack)
	sedation	yes	yes (couch-lock)

PHARMACEUTICAL DRUG	EFFECTS AND ADVERSE EFFECTS	OPIOID	CANNABIS
	Common Effects and Adverse Effects		
	respiratory depression	yes	no
	respiratory arrest	yes (dose dependent)	no
	hypotension (low blood pressure)	yes	yes
	dry mouth	yes	no
	constipation	yes	no
	constricted pupils	yes	no
	itching (pruritis)	yes	maybe (if dose too high)
	nausea/vomiting	yes	maybe (if dose too high)
	hyperalgesia	yes (dose dependent)	no (if used alone)
	fatal overdose	high risk in certain people	low risk
	addictive	yes (severe)	no physical symptoms
	withdrawal symptoms	no	yes
	red sclera (white of eye)	yes	no
	sweating	yes	yes (usually slight)
	increased heart rate	often decreases	increases (the "munchies")
	appetite	yes	no
	chronic use of opioids can reduce sex drive	yes	no
	reduced estrogen	yes	no
	reduced testosterone		
	Less Common Effects and Adverse Effects		
	serotonin syndrome	yes	no
	adrenal insufficiency	yes	no

five

Opioid Withdrawal: The Current State of Affairs and New Possibilities

Alleviating Symptoms of Opioid Withdrawal

 Opioids: possible–good[291]
Cannabinoids: possible–good[292]

ALLOW ME TO TELL another story from my paramedic days. One cold and foggy morning from the Sunset District of San Francisco, a call came about a kid who fell from the monkey bars at a playground and fractured his arm. He was crying and in great pain when we arrived. Before I was able to straighten the angulated fractures, splint them, and take him to the General Hospital trauma center, I started an intravenous line and injected a few milligrams of morphine. As I was pushing the syringe I saw his grimace relax a bit, and at the same time I couldn't help but wonder if I might be one piece in a chain of events that would contribute to getting this kid hooked on some form of opioid down the road.

It may seem far-fetched to some readers that addiction would happen to a child, but consider another example: in Kentucky alone the number of babies born drug-dependent rose 23-fold over the period of a decade

(2001–2014), with the majority of them addicted to opioids. In the majority of cases the mother was given physician-prescribed opioids (68%) or an opioid-based drug to treat opioid addiction such as methadone or buprenorphine (Suboxone) before she got pregnant.[293] This glimpse into a small slice of the population might give you an idea of how many people of all ages and both genders are becoming opioid addicts nationwide.

Each year, more and more infants are exposed in the womb to opioids, leading to babies born in withdrawal. These unfortunate infants present their distress by crying inconsolably, often with a distinct high-pitched sound, and exhibiting symptoms that include insomnia, fever, sweating, a rapid heartbeat, constant agitation or restlessness, gastrointestinal disturbances such as vomiting, lack of appetite, and diarrhea, and neurological and musculoskeletal complications that include flu-like symptoms, increased pain sensitivity, stiff body, jolts, spasms, and seizure activities. While this is certainly a dire situation, there is a silver lining: the contemporary rise in infant addiction has caused us to learn a few things about opioid addiction and withdrawal in the general population. We've already discussed in earlier chapters how intertwined pain and its treatment with opioids are for so many people.

What is the current orthodox treatment for these addicted infants? Oral opioids—drops of morphine administered by mouth in a dose that is just enough to calm them and induce some form of food cravings. After a few weeks, these tiny patients must begin their process of weaning not from the mother's breast but from the drug to which they are hooked. Well-meaning health care providers often separate the mother from the baby. Meeting the constant needs of a high number of drug-dependent babies has been challenging given the available resources. Urban hospital resources specializing in neonatal care have been overwhelmed with the sheer volume of tiny babies in distress, most of them arriving by ambulance from rural areas where appropriate facilities do not exist. A number of mostly private ambulance companies carved a niche for themselves by outfitting their units with portable incubators; they saw their business booming overall as health care costs skyrocketed. Out of necessity, compassion, or both, the search for a better way has led to a few interesting discoveries that are relevant to the topic of this book.

Researchers found that, like adults going through withdrawal, infant patients benefited from a calm, quiet, dimly lit place and, even more importantly, they significantly benefited from emotional support, connection, love, closeness, and intimacy. How did medical researchers discover that? The use of morphine to calm withdrawing babies dropped from 98 to 14 percent when the following measures were implemented: mothers received support and education in meeting the special needs of their little ones; mothers or other relatives were sleeping in the baby's room, always available, omnipresent, and attuned to the baby's needs; and when neither was present, professional consolers were substituted to hold, cuddle, and comfort the distressed infant. The result benefited not just the baby, it facilitated mother-to-child and family bonding while also lowering the hospital stay from twenty-two to about six days, which amounts to a sizable sum of health care cost savings.[294]

The takeaway? A mother informed and educated about meeting her own unique withdrawal needs and those of her infant, with a supportive environment for both, is a winning model for the future. Adult treatment models from Portugal confirm the benefits of nurturing and supportive environments that maintain connection, especially when symptoms of pain and withdrawal demand often-difficult inward attention.[295]

Cannabis for Treating Opioid Withdrawal

Selected Scientific Evidence: A Brief Review

The earliest scientific evidence that suggested engaging the endocannabinoid system in the treatment of opioid withdrawal is a study that was conducted in 1976. Researchers discovered in experiments with guinea pigs that cannabinoids may be useful in opioid detoxification. The test animals were hooked on morphine and then injected with Narcan, an opiate antidote, to artificially induce withdrawal symptoms. Scientists posited that withdrawal symptoms were mitigated by the oral administration of delta-9-THC, with test range from 1 to 10 mg/kg, via reduction of acetylcholine release in the affected tissue sites.[296]

It wasn't until 1995 that another study conducted on mice similarly suggested endocannabinoid involvement in mitigating opioid withdrawal symptoms. Mice were given increasing doses of morphine until conditioned. Once more the synthetic narcotic antagonist Narcan was injected to induce withdrawal symptoms such as twitching and weight loss. Instead of giving the test animals THC, for this study scientists injected the human body's own version, the endogenous cannabinoid anandamide, resulting in a decrease of symptoms of withdrawal, seen in the numbers of jumps and loss of body weight.[297] Anandamide binds to the same receptor sites as THC (CB1 and CB2), and as such a possible role is suggested for it and endocannabinoid engagement in cases of opioid withdrawal symptoms.

The next insights about endocannabinoid system involvement in opioid withdrawal came from a study conducted at the University of Milan in Italy in 2000, where a team of researchers coadministered the synthetic CB1 cannabinoid receptor antagonist SR141716A along with morphine to induce analgesic effects and conditioning in rats. Results showed that treatments with SR141716A did not influence the development of tolerance to the morphine analgesic effect but significantly reduced the intensity of Narcan-induced opiate withdrawal in tolerant rats, seen in a significant reduction in the number of incidents of digging, teeth chattering, and penile licking.[298] Another such study discovered that chronic but not acute administration of the CB1 antagonist SR141716A reduced opioid withdrawal symptoms in mice.[299]

Later research clarified that SR141716A (a.k.a. rimonabant) is an extremely potent CB1 receptor antagonist[300] that also acts as a direct antagonist at mu-opioid receptor sites.[301]

SR141716A was initially approved in Europe in 2006 for the treatment of obesity, but two years later was withdrawn.[302] To better understand this rather sudden change, it may help to think of it this way: THC, a mild CB1 agonist, can give you the munchies, yet it also commonly produces life-affirming euphoria. Thus a CB1 antagonist did not just suppress appetite—it also caused dysphoria in some patients in the form of severe depression and suicidal tendencies.[303]

The next preclinical experiment in the timeline was conducted at Kyushu University in Japan in 2001, where researchers examined the effects of another endocannabinoid, called 2-arachidonoylglycerol (2-AG), on Narcan-precipitated withdrawal in morphine-dependent mice. This same study also examined the effects of delta-8-THC and HU-210, a potent CB1 agonist. Results demonstrated a significant reduction in withdrawal symptoms (jumping and forepaw tremor) for 2-AG, delta-8-THC, and HU-210.[304] Later studies would reveal that HU-210 is a very potent CB1 agonist,[305] about 100 times more potent at the same receptor than THC.[306]

Later in 2001, insights from an experiment conducted on mice at the Virginia Commonwealth University began to indicate a reciprocal relationship between CB1 receptors and mu-opioid receptors in drug-dependence models.[307] This relationship was confirmed by French researchers in an experiment conducted on mice. They demonstrated that delta-9-THC induced analgesic and antidepressant effects by releasing and facilitating the effects of the body's own enkephalins (an opioid ligand). This study also showed that THC reduced opioid withdrawal symptoms without reducing reward responses. This led to the important discovery that even at high dosages and with chronic use of cannabinoids, cannabinoids did not seem to increase psychic dependence on opioids.[308] The latter finding was one of the first arrows directly aimed at the gateway theory, which holds that the use of cannabis leads to the use of stronger drugs.

By 2002 anandamide was back in the spotlight. An experiment conducted on mice showed that increased levels of the body's own version of THC, called anandamide, which binds to the same receptor sites CB1 and CB2, were able to reduce spontaneously occurring opioid withdrawal symptoms.[309] (See chapter 6 to learn about how to increase your anandamide levels naturally.)

In 2003 scientists from the Virginia Commonwealth University discovered that oral coadministration of delta-9-THC (20 mg/kg) with opioids was able to prevent opioid withdrawal symptoms and reduced oral opioid tolerance and dependence. It was the first evidence to suggest that synergistic effects between opioids and cannabinoids may provide a new mechanism allowing long-term efficacy of opioids when necessary, while potentially enhancing their safety profile by reducing the risks of developing tolerance and dependence.[310] That synergy was confirmed in another study conducted on arthritic rats in 2007. Researchers showed that coadministration of THC can enhance the analgesic effects of opioids and reduce the risk of developing opioid tolerance.[311]

The first human trial examining the potential synergistic effects of opioids and cannabis was conducted at San Francisco General Hospital in 2011. Twenty-one patients with chronic pains on a regimen of twice-daily dosages of opioids were admitted for a five-day inpatient stay. In addition to their opioid prescriptions, each was given vaporized cannabis to inhale three times a day. Results indicated a significant decrease in pain by 27 percent after the inclusion of cannabis to their regimen. The treating physician concluded that coadministration of opioids and cannabinoids may allow opioid treatments at lower dosages while reducing the risk of adverse effects.[312]

You may remember from chapter 4 that neuropathic pains are notoriously difficult to treat. First-line drug recommendations include antidepressants and anticonvulsant drugs, with opioids recommended as a second-line approach. An evidentiary analysis published in 2012 suggested that physicians who treat central or peripheral neuropathic pain with second-line recommendations of opioids ought to prescribe cannabis use prior to opioid consumption for potentially better analgesic effects and as a harm-reduction measure.[313] A meta-analysis published in 2013 confirmed several potential mechanisms through which cannabinoids may prevent opiate dependence and ease withdrawal,[314] adding more gravitas to developing cannabis-inclusive protocols.

You may have seen the news. In 2014 potent evidence emerged clearly demonstrating that new medical cannabis laws were in direct relationship to significantly lower opioid overdose mortality rates. Hundreds if not thousands of people annually who might have died from opioid overdoses to treat chronic pain were still alive.[315] Let that sink in for a moment. The results were confirmed in a later small-size trial conducted on cannabis-using patients. Among several of their findings, researchers reported a declining concurrent use of opioids by 42 percent.[316]

Emerging Evidence Paints a More Complex and Holistic Picture

It can be argued that the quality of our emotions defines the quality of our lives. Emotions have a specific role in motivation and behavior that is especially relevant to addiction, including propensities for pleasure seeking and pain avoidance. Emotional states have molecular counterparts—for example, epinephrine is associated with fear or excitement, cortisol with stress, and anandamide with ease. It is noteworthy that many of the neurotransmitters, communication molecules, hormones, and pro- and anti-inflammatory cytokines, as well as their mental-emotional correlates, are either partly or significantly modulated by the endocannabinoid system. (Chapter 6 looks at these dynamics more closely.)

In 2015, in a study titled "The Dark Side of Emotion: The Addiction Perspective," the author implicates the body's own cannabinoids in the modulation of emotions and posits that endocannabinoids may play a protective role in preventing drug dependence.[317] This brings us to another relevant cannabinoid, namely cannabidiol (CBD), as a potential treatment for various symptoms relevant to opioid addiction and withdrawal. For instance, CBD has proven abilities to reduce dysphoric states such as depression[318] and anxiety,[319] as well as psychotic symptoms.[320] CBD is a potent neuroprotective,[321] antispasmodic, and antiseizure agent,[322] and as such may be relevant to treating withdrawal-related increased sensitivities to pain, muscle cramps, and involuntary movements, respectively. CBD reduces stress and autonomic responses to stress such as elevated heart rate, which may also be therapeutically relevant.[323] It has significant anti-inflammatory abilities[324] that may play a role in mitigating gastrointestinal pain and diarrhea[325] and inflammation-based joint pain.[326]

The orthodox medical community is slowly beginning to consider the use of cannabinoids in the treatment of opioid withdrawal symptoms. For instance, a review published in 2015 by an international team of researchers concluded that the data suggest a strong foundation for further exploration of CBD as a therapeutic intervention against opioid addiction and relapse.[327] Authors of another review, in 2016, based their findings on emerging efforts to engage the endocannabinoid system in the treatment of opioid addiction. Among the supporting findings was a discovery related to the enzyme that degrades anandamide, the body's own version of THC. When inhibitors were used to prevent the breakdown of anandamide and thus increase its bioavailability in the bodies of rodents, it produced a clear reduction in opioid withdrawal symptoms.[328]

By 2017 a study conducted on 2,897 cannabis-using patients, with more than a third of them having used opioid analgesia in the preceding six months, by researchers from the University of California at Berkeley, Kent State, and WebMD, noted that:

> Respondents overwhelmingly reported that cannabis provided relief on par with their other medications, but without the unwanted side effects. Ninety-seven percent of the sample "strongly agreed/agreed" that they are able to decrease the amounts of opiates they consume when they also use cannabis, and 81 percent "strongly agreed/agreed" that taking cannabis by itself was more effective at treating their condition than taking cannabis with opioids. Results were similar for those using cannabis with nonopioid-based pain medications.[329]

The emerging evidence is clearly shifting toward the cannabinoid health sciences in providing patients dealing with pain and opioid withdrawal symptoms a novel possibility for effective, less expensive, more natural, and safer alternatives. This view is further supported by the results of another experiment, published in 2017, conducted on mice, which found that CBD (10 mg/kg) blocked opioid reward and as such may be useful in addiction treatments.[330]

I'd like to close this section with a quote from Jasmin L. Hurd, author of a 2017 study published in the journal *Trends in Neurosciences*:

> Epidemics require a paradigm shift in thinking about all possible solutions. The rapidly changing sociopolitical marijuana landscape provides a foundation for the therapeutic development of medicinal cannabidiol to address the current opioid abuse crisis.[331]

Review Summary: Taken together, the results of studies reported in this chapter show that all three cannabinoids discussed in this book—anandamide, THC, and CBD—have demonstrated potent therapeutic abilities in alleviating opioid withdrawal symptoms. A variety of different mechanisms underlie these abilities, as presented in chapters 3 and 6.

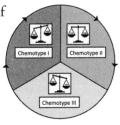

For some, a typical approach combining cannabinoid therapies with a mind-body approach might start with the need for a THC-rich chemotype-I of cannabis or cannabis-containing product to produce analgesic effects in the treatment of pain or in mitigating the pain of withdrawal symptoms. The idea here would be to slowly but surely move clockwise as depicted in the above graphic. As symptoms are managed, you may want to include more CBD in your regimen by utilizing a chemotype II with a relative equal ratio of THC and CBD. If the relief you need is holding, continue the shift to the right, to where you will be leaning on a chemotype-III cannabis flower or cannabis-containing product. Another person might prefer or need to start right away with a chemotype-III. As your body and mind begin to rebalance your neurotransmitter profiles and solidify your healing process, you might be able to complete your course of cannabis treatment and solely rely of emotional self-regulation strategies to maintain flow and balance of your communication molecules and their emotional associates.

If you need more information about specific symptoms such as anxiety, depression, or spasms and which cannabis chemotype might provide you with the best possible relief, you may want have a closer look at the individual studies noted in this chapter.

six

The Endocannabinoid System and Its Role in Returning Balance to Body, Mind, and Emotions

GIVEN THE EMERGING EVIDENCE, one could speculate that if the prime use of opium is to replace all ill feelings with temporary analgesic euphoria, then the prime directive of cannabis in remedying opiate abuse is to restore and maintain balance. It appears that in addition to its synergistic boosting effect with opiate use[332]—allowing smaller doses for the same relief when combining cannabis with opiates—cannabis mitigates the pain of opiate withdrawal via numerous mechanisms (outlined in chapter 5) and as such may also help some opiate users avoid becoming addicted in the first place.

In previous chapters we examined how and what type of cannabis can support what type of pain relief. In this chapter we look at the potential negative impact of opioids and opioid withdrawal on specific neurotransmitters, hormones, signaling proteins, and other communication molecules and their associated emotions, and how the endocannabinoid system (ECS) works to return both molecules and emotions to a more balanced state and sustain that state. You may find this chapter of special interest if you are one of those individuals who is really interested in taking more agency in your healing process.

Opioid use as well as opioid withdrawal symptoms can significantly alter the balance of a great variety of neurotransmitters, often in an inverse relationship. With this comes an imbalance in the associated mental-emotional qualities or functions. Resulting imbalances underlie physical and psychological opioid withdrawal.

Allow me, for starters, to offer some simplified examples using single emotions and some of the neurotransmitter molecules commonly associated with them to demonstrate their interconnectivity. For instance, during times of stress, cortisol and epinephrine levels rise. When we are depressed, our serotonin and dopamine levels become depleted. And, when we are in love, we are flooded in oxytocin, dopamine, and serotonin.

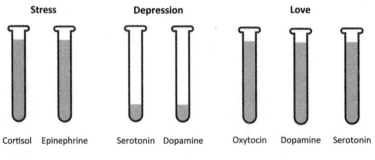

Figure 6.1.

Indeed, neurotransmitters and corresponding emotions function like traffic on a two-way street, with the ECS modulating (directing, balancing), either in part or significantly, the flow of traffic. Homeostasis (balance) is its prime purpose.

Let's use adrenaline (epinephrine) to look more specifically at how this process is thought to work. Epinephrine is a hormone and neurotransmitter produced by the adrenal glands located on top of each kidney. It is associated with fight, flight, or freeze responses. Epinephrine increases heart rate and raises blood pressure, but at the same time it relaxes the smooth muscles of the airways, facilitating increased oxygen demands necessary in any life-or-death situation. Psychologically the hormone is clearly associated with emotions such as fear. Now the two-way-street part: Healthy students were injected with either epinephrine or saltwater and were shown the same movie clips. Those injected with the hormone responded with greater fear and emotional intensity when confronted by a scary scene than the placebo-injected control group.[333]

ECS participates in the modulation of this neurotransmitter via the adrenal glands, which are richly endowed with CB1 receptor sites.[334] And while pain and opioid withdrawal symptoms tend to increase epinephrine release, preclinical trials show that CB1 receptor activation seems to reduce this as well as other fight, flight, or freeze molecules,[335] and as such may provide much-needed relief from the stress of pain or withdrawal.

The hypothesis is further supported by an experiment conducted on humans. Researchers discovered that after inducing a coma (via barbiturates) and injecting Narcan (opioid antidote) to instantly force the body to go into withdrawal while letting opioid-addicted patients sleep through the worst of their symptoms produced a thirty-fold increase in epinephrine, and with it a significant rise in heart rate and blood pressure. The finding suggests the possibility that long-term opioid use reduces sympathoadrenal and cardiovascular function, which is acutely reversed by mu-opioid receptor blockade, causing a sudden withdrawal.[336] It seems like the body can't be tricked into skipping the step of facing dysphoria on the road to recovery.

As we have seen with the example of adrenaline (epinephrine), the ECS modulates a number of other relevant neurotransmitters toward balance in body, mind, and emotions. Here is what a broader but typical neurotransmitter profile might look like at various stages of opioid withdrawal (not a complete list).

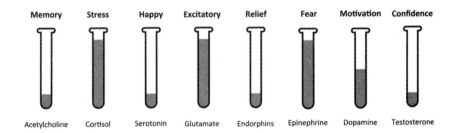

Figure 6.2. Typical neurotransmitter profile under stressful conditions

Forging New Neuronal Pathways

The proper type of cannabis matched to one's specific needs and preferences can create a therapeutic shift in molecules but also a shift in the normal state of awareness that makes it easier to accept oneself, especially in the presence of otherwise intolerable feeling or emotions.

As you will see shortly, what is true for the properly dosed cannabis experience is also true for emotional authenticity, where all emotions are felt and released. When feeling and experiencing all emotions—both constricting and expansive ones—without attachment or reservation, neurotransmitter profiles quickly adjust, fluctuate, and flow from moment to moment, releasing blockages, flushing pockets of resistance, and rapidly contributing to building new neuronal pathways in the brain.

Together with these changes comes the possibility of new narrative, new options, and healthier choices. Indeed, just facing and accepting emotions will often cause a shift of energy, almost always in a positive direction. The point here is to know that the positive effects of cannabis on body and mind are achieved via chemical changes that can be induced *without* cannabis when you understand the process. So, how does it work?

Let's start this way: synapses that fire together wire together. A synapse (more specifically a synaptic cleft) is empty space (a gateway) between nerve cells. This is true for the entire brain and for all those superhighways of connection we call our nervous system. When we touch a toe to the cool surface of a pond, the sensation is transmitted from one nerve cell to another in the form of electrical signals that travel up the nerves until they reach a synapse. The signal (the charge) must now cross the gateway (the synaptic cleft), and it does so by releasing chemicals (neurotransmitters) into the space between nerve cells. It is upon these that the electrical charge rides across the portal and continues its journey to the brain where the signal is received and processed, and where we get to choose how we will respond. Stop? Pull back? Jump in? We decide. Nerve impulses, composed and initiated by our responding thoughts, feelings, and chemicals, travel through the body on nerve pathways and across synaptic clefts and induce muscles to react accordingly.

Here is what's instructive: the body is hardwired for efficiency. For every time the same charge is expressed, the gateways grow closer to reduce distance and make it easier for the electrical charge to cross the cleft. The more often we think the same thought, experience the same feeling, tell ourselves the same story, the easier it will be to redo it until it becomes the path of least resistance. Our repeated thoughts and our repeated responses are some of the most powerful forces that shape our brain and our entire nervous system, and in doing so, for better or worse, have great power over our health and well-being. We are designed to do this all the time. Our brain organizes, reorganizes, grows, evolves, or devolves with every thought we think, especially those we think more frequently. Our most repeated thoughts and emotional narratives become the basis for how we experience ourselves, others, and the world around us.

Let's apply this to opioid withdrawal. The euphoria wears off, slowly at first. Initially we may think, "This is OK. I can deal with this." However, it doesn't take long until we generate our first signal, the first nagging thought, the first anticipation of what will surely come around the next bend of our experience. Sooner than we'd like, the anticipation becomes anxiety, which quickly turns into the same confrontation with the emotional material that must not be named, that must be hidden at all cost. Sure enough, there it is, we recall a memory of how bad it was the last time. The thought, the memory, the belief induces the feeling, and we are faced with the same dysphoria, the same withdrawal experience, only worse. We reach for the emotional self-regulation strategy we are familiar with—we reach for a new patch of fentanyl, and in short order the opioids do their job. Euphoria kicks in as the pain and discomfort become a quickly fading echo of the past. And, for a few precious hours, we are OK. In opioid withdrawal, that is a common signal pathway of least resistance, or the synaptic pathway most traveled. As a result, natural emotional processing is suppressed and replaced by external opioid-based emotional designs, creating the desired but temporary emotional experience of analgesic euphoria.

For far too many people who opt for emotional authorship (self-regulation) via an opioid, the price extracted is neurochemical imbalances that find a crescendo in the dysphoria of withdrawal symptoms. However, there are other, healthier emotional self-regulation strategies we can consider and realize by the exact same mechanism.

Knowing what emotions are associated with what type of molecule allows us to better engage in constructive and therapeutic emotional self-regulation strategies. In this way, we can more consciously turn a severely blocked and stressed neurotransmitter environment into one that is free-flowing and balanced. Developing emotional authenticity as a self-regulation strategy, for example, also produces psychological resilience that is able to better respond to any stressor, including debilitating withdrawal-based dysphoria.

Instead of running from dysphoric states, we are able to summon the resources to be in the presence of difficult emotional material without recoil. Instead of chronically evading the anticipated difficult thoughts or feelings, we tap into the capacity to embrace them or even learn from them, for example, what's their point of origin, their purpose, or how to transcend them?

In contrast to the tendency of opioids to blunt all difficult emotions by creating a single focus on analgesic euphoria, a properly dosed cannabis experience or an effective mind-body technique can create a similarly deeply relaxed state of mind that can alter our physiology and our state of consciousness in such a way as to enable us to be with otherwise intolerable emotional material. Empowered by profound human resources we all have access to, such as the capacity for healing, awareness, and mindfulness, it is easier to take the often challenging but necessary steps not just to face dysphoria but to set the stage to answer the demand for change called for in the intensity and depth of pain of our withdrawal.

The following graphic includes a list of neurotransmitters and other communication molecules and their emotional associates (modulated, either in part or significantly, by the ECS) that are commonly blocked, diminished, and disrupted by inappropriate opioid use and during times of withdrawal (see the checkmarks).

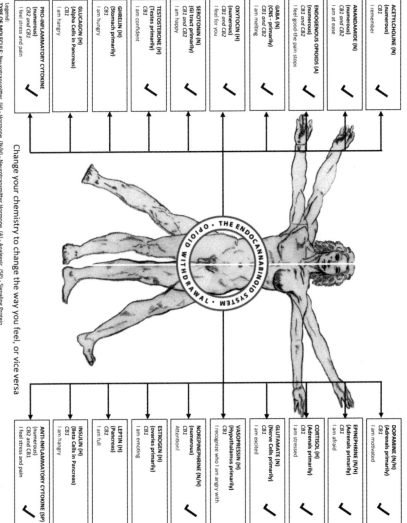

Figure 6.3. Neurotransmitters affected by opioid use and withdrawal

ACETYLCHOLINE (N)
(numerous)
CB1
I remember

ANANDAMIDE (N)
(numerous)
CB1 and CB2
I am at ease

ENDOGENOUS OPIOIDS (A)
(numerous)
CB1 and CB2
I feel good-the pain stops

GABA (N)
(CNS - primarily)
CB1 and CB2
I am melting

OXYTOCIN (H)
(numerous)
CB1 and CB2
I feel for you

SEROTONIN (N)
(GI tract primarily)
CB1 and CB2
I am happy

TESTOSTERONE (H)
(Testes primarily)
CB1
I am confident

GHRELIN (H)
(Stomach primarily)
CB1
I am hungry

GLUCAGON (H)
(Alpha Cells in Pancreas)
CB1
I am hungry

PRO-INFLAMMATORY CYTOKINE
(numerous)
CB2 and CB1
I feel stress and pain

Change your chemistry to change the way you feel, or vice versa

THE ENDOCANNABINOID SYSTEM · OPIOID · WITHDRAWAL

DOPAMINE (N/H)
(Adrenals primarily)
CB1
I am motivated

EPINEPHRINE (N/H)
(Adrenals primarily)
CB1
I am afraid

CORTISOL (H)
(Adrenals primarily)
CB1
I am stressed

GLUTAMATE (N)
(Nerve Cells primarily)
CB1
I am excited

VASOPRESSIN (H)
(Hypothalamus primarily)
CB1
I recognize who I am angry with

NOREPHEPHRINE (N/H)
(numerous)
CB1
Attention!

ESTROGEN (H)
(ovaries primarily)
CB1
I am emoting

LEPTIN (H)
(Pancreas)
CB1
I am full

INSULIN (H)
(Beta Cells in Pancreas)
CB1
I am hungry

ANTI-INFLAMMATORY CYTOKINE (SP)
(numerous)
CB2 and CB1
I feel stress and pain

Legend:
TYPE OF MOLECULE: Neurotransmitter, (H) - Hormone, (N/H) - Neurotransmitter Hormone, (A) - Analgesic, (SP) - Signaling Protein
(Produced where): primary production location or numerous locations
Endocannabinoid receptors that modulate this molecule: CB1, CB2, or both
Corresponding emotion(s) or mental function(s) which may modulate this molecule and vis versa

SUMMARY KEY RESULTS OF SELECTED STUDIES: ECS-MODULATED NEUROTRANSMITTERS RELEVANT TO OPIOID USE AND WITHDRAWAL

Research reveals that opioid use adversely affects levels of many chemicals that balance the body's functions and moods. This short list addresses some of the more important neurotransmitters in the body, but it is not exhaustive. The notes contain the studies' published sources for readers who want more information.

Acetylcholine: Opioids decrease and inhibit acetylcholine release.[337]

Anandamide: Mitigates opioid withdrawal symptoms.[338]

Endorphins: Endogenous opioids and their receptors are modified as addiction develops.[339]

GABA: GABA receptors are involved in the control of opioid withdrawal symptoms.[340]

Oxytocin: May produce direct antiaddictive effects.[341]

Serotonin: Levels may increase during acute opioid use and may drop with chronic use.[342]

Testosterone: Research suggests suppressed level in males who chronically use opioids.[343]

Pro-inflammatory cytokines: Increase during opioid addiction and withdrawal.[344]

Dopamine: Significantly associated with the beginning of the cycle of addiction.[345]

Epinephrine: Long-term opioid use reduces sympathoadrenal function.[346]

Cortisol: Chronic opioid use suppresses cortisol levels,[347] but during withdrawal cortisol increases.[348]

Glutamate: Chronic use of opioids increases its excitatory effects.[349]

Norepinephrine: Likely to be elevated during acute withdrawal from chronic opioid use.[350]

Strategies for Enhancing or Balancing ECS-Modulated Molecules Relevant to Opioid Withdrawal

The idea here is to prevent blockages by allowing a constant flow of natural expansion and constriction. Each and all of these molecules and their associated emotions are a necessity for the human experience.

There will always be negative (constricting) and positive (expansive) feelings and emotions. However, what creates resilience in the face of adversity, stress, or a potential trigger is to recognize that none will last forever, and to develop the skill sets that allows you to reduce any tendencies for negative emotions and replace them with tendencies for positive ones.

For your consideration, here are some practical suggestions for emotional self-regulation strategies that might be therapeutically helpful in assisting your endocannabinoid system to balance neurotransmitter profiles. The suggested strategies aim to undo blockages, reestablish balances, and create a natural sense of waxing and waning of emotional material. More specifically, the idea here is to release, reduce, or balance molecules associated with constricting emotions such as fear, stress, pain, irritation, dysphoria, or withdrawal, such as epinephrine, cortisol, norepinephrine, dopamine, glutamate, and pro-inflammatory cytokines. At the same time, the suggested strategies aim to enhance or balance molecules associated with expansive mental activity and emotions, such as learning (acetylcholine), bliss (anandamide), euphoria (endorphins), relaxation (GABA), empathy (oxytocin), happiness (serotonin), and well-being (anti-inflammatory cytokines).

Acetylcholine

Associated with learning, memory, plasticity, arousal, attention, and reward, acetylcholine is produced by nerve cells (neurons) throughout the human body. It is a naturally occurring neurotransmitter of the autonomic nervous system and the only neurotransmitter of the voluntary nervous system. As such, acetylcholine may be involved in creativity and the ability to enjoy life's pleasures and passions. It may enhance our capacity for learning and remembering.

Reduced acetylcholine levels are associated with insomnia, impaired creativity, and dementia in Alzheimer's patients. Research has shown that opioids decrease and inhibit acetylcholine release.[351]

Nerve cells express endocannabinoid receptors. A low to medium dose of THC can increase acetylcholine in the brain, while a high dose of THC may lower it (an effect not confirmed in human trials);[352] this indicates a potential balancing role of the ECS. To boost or balance your acetylcholine availability:

- Learn and use a new word every day.

- Meditate to enhance focus and concentration.

- Improve your memory with crossword puzzles, riddles, and so on.

- Recall a rare emotion in detail until you feel it.

- Think of a feeling you never had and imagine what it feels like.

Anandamide

This endocannabinoid is produced in cell membranes (containing CB1 and CB2 receptors). It is the body's own version of THC and is associated with emotions such as bliss, social connection,[353] and gentle euphoria—think "runner's high."[354] When anandamide binds with CB1 and CB2, it produces similar effects to THC but with less intensity. Cannabidiol (CBD) reduces the enzyme that breaks down anandamide, making it more bioavailable and thus inducing CB1- and CB2-activated analgesic, relaxing, and mood-elevating effects with a wide therapeutic window, reducing the potential for any adverse effects sometimes associated with THC.

Anandamide mitigates opioid withdrawal symptoms[355] and may also reduce high blood pressure, fear, depression, and anxiety[356] and can initiate analgesic effects.[357] Thus it is likely helpful in a variety of opioid withdrawal symptoms. To boost or balance your anandamide availability:

- Exercise such as high-intensity endurance running significantly increased anandamide and runner's high.[358]

- Meaningful social interactions may increase anandamide levels naturally.
- Meditation practices may increase anandamide levels naturally.

Endogenous Opioids (Endorphins)

Endorphins are produced by cells of the central nervous system and in the pituitary gland. One of the more significant keys to balancing your emotional tone naturally as well as to killing pain and shifting energy, endorphins are the body's own opium. Endogenous opioids bind with opiate receptors to reduce stress and pain perceptions; they may also play a role interpersonal relationships and appetite.

Associated emotions include euphoria, elation, and relief from pain. THC can modulate the release of endogenous opioids,[359] and CBD is considered a very promising agent in the cotreatment of pain in conjunction with opioids. Research conducted on animals has shown that both CBD and to a lesser degree THC (6 times less than CBD) bind noncompetitively with mu and delta opioid receptors and as such can boost opioid-based analgesic effects, allowing for lower doses that are effective while reducing the risk of addiction and overdose.[360]

Endogenous opioids and their receptors are modified as addiction develops.[361] To boost or balance your endorphin availability:

- Strenuous exercise
- A pleasurable massage
- A deeply relaxing acupuncture session
- Intimacy and sex
- Inducing deep relaxation response via cannabis or relaxation technique

GABA (Gamma Aminobutyric Acid)

This amino acid is produced by the brain when it breaks down the excitatory neurotransmitter glutamate. GABA produces a calming and relaxing effect on nerve cells and muscle tone. When GABA and glutamate balance each other, relaxation and excitement balance each other, and vice versa. Endocannabinoid interaction with GABA is complex and to date a poorly understood subject.

GABA receptors are involved in the control of opioid withdrawal symptoms.[362] GABA reduces fear signaling in the amygdala,[363] and low levels of GABA may produce irritability, insomnia, anxiety, depression, panic attacks, lack of empathy, aggression, antisocial behavior, a craving for carbohydrates, and adrenal fatigue. Endocannabinoids can modulate the release of GABA and glutamate in various portions of the brain.[364] To boost or balance your GABA availability:

- Yoga sessions increased brain GABA level by 27 percent.[365]
- Regular exercise increases GABA level.[366]
- Meditation practices have shown to enhance GABA levels.[367]

Oxytocin

This hormone is produced by both genders in the hypothalamus and stored by the pituitary gland. It is largely noticed in its involvement in female reproduction, inducing birth as well as mother-child bonding. Evidence suggests that oxytocin may produce direct antiaddiction effects.[368] Opioid withdrawal can overexcite oxytocin neurons, producing an increase in oxytocin brain and plasma levels. Higher withdrawal stress levels mean higher plasma oxytocin levels,[369] a potential response by the body to mitigate stress. Oxytocin has shown to inhibit morphine tolerance and to mitigate opioid-based withdrawal symptoms.[370] To boost or balance your oxytocin availability:

- Sex[371]
- Orgasm[372]
- Closeness, tenderness, intimacy[373]
- Trust[374]
- Generosity[375]

However, oxytocin has a short half-life, and therefore its effects last only a few minutes,[376] which suggests that to maximize the potential health benefits of oxytocin, we need to keep our focus on generating these qualities. A recent study discovered a significant connection in oxytocin-initiated anandamide CB1 signaling producing the experience of social rewards or pleasure.[377]

Serotonin

Serotonin is primarily produced in the gut. Endocannabinoid CB2 receptors are also abundantly present in the intestinal environment. Only a limited amount of research exists to date examining serotonin signaling during acute opiate withdrawal. However, some animal studies conducted on rodents suggest that serotonin levels increase during acute opioid use.[378] The effects of chronic opioid uses on serotonin levels is still a subject of debate. For instance, an examination of brains from deceased heroin users suggested that serotonin activity may be reduced after prolonged use.[379]

Studies have shown that your mood affects your serotonin levels. As such, developing habits for positive emotion and reducing habits that produce negative affect raises and lower your serotonin levels naturally.[380] The endocannabinoid-induced modulation of stress-related disorders such as anxieties or depression appears to be mediated, at least in part, through the regulation of the serotoninergic system.[381] To boost or balance your serotonin availability:

- Reduce toxic stress (chronic stress reduces serotonin).
- Appropriately express and release constricting emotions.
- Be Happy! Merely remembering happy situations and memories gives you a boost. Also, happiness tends to occur naturally when you meet your basic human needs for safety, security, pleasure, and belonging.
- Get a massage to boost your happiness and your serotonin.
- Exercise increases serotonin production and release.
- Balanced exposure to sunlight increases vitamin D, which is involved in promoting serotonin production.

Epinephrine (Adrenaline)

Associated with fear, excitement, anxiety, and stress, adrenaline is produced in the adrenal glands, which are located on top of each kidney. These glands are richly endowed with CB1 receptor sites. It is a hormone and neurotransmitter associated with fight, flight, or freeze responses as well as the long-term memory of intense events. It is instantly released in the presence of anything that scares or threatens us in some way. While it comes on near instantaneously, it takes a few minutes to break down. To reduce or balance your epinephrine levels:

Slow down: studies have shown that when we are afraid, we limit our choices and close down to many otherwise possible responses. Fear, like most of the constricting emotions, such as anxiety, anger, defensiveness, flourishes with the speed of thought and speech. In other words, the more dangerous the tigers you imagine, the more your mind will try to protect you by rapidly trying to find a safe place to hide. We think fast and we speak fast. However, a person in constant fear tends to always imagine more tigers. Slow down your thinking. It is your imagination; it does not belong to fear. Take it back and go slow-motion in your mind's eye. Slow down your speech. In conversation, speak one or two sentences, then take a break and breathe, relax, and listen to the response. Repeat. Any relaxation technique of your choice, appropriate exercise, or mindfulness practice can provide you with similar calming results.

Cortisol

Associated with stress, fear, anxiety, restlessness, shame, guilt, low self-esteem, and low self-worth, cortisol is a stress hormone, and like epinephrine is produced by the adrenal gland with an abundant supply of CB1 receptor sites. The presence of corticosteroids stimulates the body's production of anandamide, which may account for the way in which anandamide influences the antidepressant effects of exercise.[382]

Chronic opioid use suppresses the human hypothalamic-pituitary-adrenal axis, producing significantly lower cortisol levels than controls.[383] During opioid withdrawal, cortisol increases and reflects the severity of withdrawal symptoms.[384] A double-blind, placebo-controlled trial conducted on heroin-dependent patients suggested a more complex role of cortisol in craving. Results showed that a single dose of 20 mg of cortisol reduced cravings in low-dose heroin users but not in medium- or high-dose users.[385] A study conducted on heroin-dependent individuals beyond the five-day acute withdrawal phase discovered that cortisol levels are elevated at night when compared to healthy controls.[386] To balance your cortisol levels:

Balancing cortisol levels and its mental-emotional correlates may require time and effort. For instance, an experiment conducted at the University of California suggests a connection between the emotions of shame and guilt and the psychological constructs of self-worth and self-esteem. People burdened with shame and those with low self-esteem and a low sense of self-worth exhibited increased levels of cortisol when compared to a random control group.[387]

Norepinephrine

Associated with attention, excitement, alertness, urgency, concentration, focus, and motivation, noradrenalin is primarily produced by the adrenal gland. Interactivity between noradrenalin releases is demonstrated by an experiment that discovered that GABA, THC, and anandamide inhibit norepinephrine levels.[388]

While only a limited number of studies have examined the effects of norepinephrine during opioid withdrawal, those that do exist suggest that norepinephrine signaling will be affected and is likely to be elevated during acute withdrawal from chronic opioid use.[389] To reduce or balance your epinephrine levels:

Use logic to analyze your fear. Determine if your fear is keeping you from real danger or if it is mainly a projection of a fear-fueled imagination or memory. For instance, are you standing at the edge of a cliff, and your fear is asking you to step back to safety? Or is your fear telling you that love is for fools because your first date as a teenager didn't go so well?

Dopamine

Dopamine is associated with motivation, reward, arousal, emotional processing, and memory. While dopamine is produced by the adrenal glands, the larger dopamine neurotransmitter system is associated and key to the beginning of the cycle of addiction—regulating reward-related mental and emotional expressions such as pleasure, cognition, emotion, and motivation. On the other hand, the neurotransmitter glutamate is associated with completing the cycle of addiction by promoting compulsivity and diminished control.[390]

Research conducted on rodents found that opioid withdrawal affected dopamine release.[391] Lack of dopamine is associated with fatigue, failure to complete tasks, low libido, and burdensome emotional memories. Endocannabinoids modulate a number of neurotransmitters that are involved in many physiological processes relevant to addiction, among them dopamine.[392] To boost or balance your dopamine availability:

- Listen to music that accesses and moves deep emotions.[393]

- Meditation induces changes of consciousness by modulating dopamine tone.[394]

Glutamate

Glutamate is associated with excitatory sensations and "upper" effects. Too much glutamate is toxic to nerve cells and a contributing factor in common withdrawal symptoms such as insomnia, restlessness, or anxiety. Glutamate is most likely produced by the mitochondria of certain brain cells (astroglia). Astroglia contain both CB1 and CB2 receptor sites. CBD and THC are able to protect cells from toxic levels of excitatory glutamate.[395]

Chronic use of opioids alters glutamate transporter levels[396] and increases its excitatory effects.[397] Opioid withdrawal increases glutamate bioavailability in the portion of the brain[398] involved in processing stress and panic, the locus coeruleus. To reduce or balance your glutamate availability:

- Reduce or cease using foods that contain glutamate.

- Reduce fear, worry, and stress with any technique of your choice (see "Epinephrine" and "Nornephrine," above).

- CBD and THC are able to protect cells from toxic levels of excitatory glutamate.[399]

Testosterone

Testosterone is produced by the gonads of both genders—the ovaries in women and the testes in males. The endocannabinoid system is involved in the modulation of sex related activities,[400] including that of sex hormones such as testosterone.[401] Both CB1 and CB2 receptor sites are found in sperm cells.[402] While anandamide is recognized as playing a modulating and necessary role in male reproduction, studies that examined the effects of plant-based cannabinoids have found mixed results. That is, some have shown that cannabis use reduces testosterone,[403] while other show no changes compared to noncannabis using males.[404]

While the effects of opioids on the hormone testosterone are poorly understood and studied, it is recognized that opioids induce their effects via the hypothalamic-pituitary-gonadal axis.[405] In general, research suggests that testosterone level is suppressed in males who chronically use opioids,[406] and they often experience a lower sex drive and less overall energy and motivation. Research into testosterone levels during withdrawal is wanting. To boost or balance testosterone:

One study discovered that about forty-five minutes to an hour of strength training increased testosterone levels regardless of age, but not to the same degree.[407]

Pro-inflammatory Cytokines

Both pro- and anti-inflammatory cytokines are signaling proteins involved in the inflammatory process. Cytokines are part of the immune system and are primarily produced by a variety of immune cells that are also richly endowed by CB2 receptor sites. As such, cytokine release is either partly or significantly modulated by the endocannabinoid system, with a focus of balance or homeostasis between pro- and anti-inflammatory types of cells.[408]

In general, research on rodents suggests that opioid-addicted rats are more vulnerable to developing inflammation,[409] and that chronic morphine exposure can induce pro-inflammatory cytokines in specific sites of the brain.[410] Specifically, two studies discovered that opioid withdrawal increases the presence of pro-inflammatory cytokines.[411] To balance pro- and anti-inflammatory cytokines:

Dietary consideration, including plant-based constituents such as terpenes or flavonoids, can play a significant role in balancing inflammatory cytokine profiles.[412] See "Inflammatory Pain" in chapter 4 for more information about which cannabinoids to consider to balance inflammatory responses. Mindfulness-based stress reduction programs have been demonstrated to reduce both loneliness and pro-inflammatory gene expression in older adults.[413] This study would also suggest that when we foster meaningful connection, we also fortify or mitigate inflammatory responses.

seven

Determining Vulnerabilities to Addiction and Developing Effective Means of Shoring Up One's Defenses

IN THE ONGOING SEARCH for causes of opioid addiction and a better understanding of its complex mechanism, different schools of thought have emerged about what constitutes the particular vulnerabilities that make one person more susceptible and another more resilient. Orthodox medicine usually focuses on three commonly agreed-upon variables, consisting of hereditary (it's your genes), environment (deviant peers, heroin chic), and the repeated use of the substance (opioid prescriptions, self-medicating). However, reality is a lot more complex, intricate, and interesting, because as we explore the broader set of contributing factors (epigenetics, mind-body relation, social trauma), novel solutions can emerge that make a real and practical difference not just to the individual but also to society at large.

Some of the vulnerabilities noted in this chapter (stress, unresolved mental-emotional pain, alienation) may or may not all apply to you, and the list is not exhaustive. Some contributors to vulnerability are big issues that require time and collective changes, while others are subject to individual interventions. For some users a single vulnerability may be enough to cross the bridge to an opioid use disorder, while for others it may take more factors or the perfect storm of all of them. Regardless of individual susceptibility, the more we know about potential vulnerabilities and how they relate to us personally, the easier it will be to take countermeasures and develop strategies and effective means to shore up defenses, thus increasing our capacity for resilience during times of opioid use.

Stress

Especially acute episodes or **stress** of a chronic nature can have a significant negative impact on our health and constitute a major vulnerability to consider in cases of opioid use disorders. Stress and drugs of abuse tend to have overlapping mechanisms.[414] The previous chapter explored how opioid use negatively affects neurotransmitter release via the hypothalamic-pituitary-adrenal (HPA) axis.[415] At the same time, the HPA axis is the body's primary stress-response mechanism.[416]

The health-eroding impact of stress starts in the womb. **Prenatal stress** (then perinatal, and stress in the early developing stage) is perhaps the first chronological vulnerability in people's lives.[417] Abundant evidence exists to show that exposure during pregnancy and early life to significant (intense or prolonged) physical, mental, and emotional stress can have effects that may persist for a lifetime, including an increased addiction risk.[418]

Stress activates fight, flight, and freeze responses via communication molecules such as epinephrine, norepinephrine, cortisol, vasopressin, and endorphins. And while these molecules are part of a natural mechanism of managing stress at any stage in life, significant prenatal stress (before birth), perinatal stress (around birth), or intense or chronic stress in the early developing years (especially before two years of age) can set the stage for a lifetime of elevated stress responses, also known as hyperreactivity. A chronic state of fight, flight, or freeze responses is the result of a hypersensitized amygdala (fear-processing center), decreased hippocampal ability (disruption of the glucocorticoid negative feedback system) to reduce stress hormone levels,[419] and diminishing dopamine release in the part of the brain (mesocorticolimbic region) that is involved in experiencing reward and addiction.

Chronic stress or episodes of acute stress continue to be major contributing vulnerabilities to developing addictive behavior, such as opioid use disorders,[420] and it may also be a cofactor for conditions that commonly share neuro-inflammation and heightened sensitivity, such as PTSD, autism, and ADHD. It may surprise you to learn that we actually have a lot of options to choose from to reduce these impacts. Although a thorough examination of the possibilities for constructively preventing and mitigating damage by prenatal stressors and the trauma of birth is beyond the scope of this book, I would like to mention at least three useful resources by scholars on the topic.

The psychiatrist Stanislav Grof conducted decades-long research into extraordinary states of consciousness using LSD and, later, holotropic breath work. He delineated a number of correlations between stressful experiences while in the womb or during the birth process itself and the later onset of chronic debilitating physical, mental, and emotional problems, including that of substance abuse. His work and suggestions about what can be done therapeutically have withstood the test of time and can be learned and employed to make a practical and long-lasting difference. See the note for suggested reading on this topic.[421]

A second resource along these lines is the work of French obstetrician Frederick Leboyer, who developed a simple method for reducing the all-too-common but preventable trauma of birth and thereby facilitating new life entering the world without the drama and trauma, without the terror, the pain, and the confusion so commonly associated with orthodox birth practices. His simple suggestions include immersing the newly born infant into a bath of body-temperature warm water, the dimming of otherwise bright operating room lights, and keeping the baby with the mother rather than giving a slap on the butt and immediately separating the baby in another room for blood tests. His book *Birth without Violence* has made a significant impact that can be seen by a great number of hospitals having implemented many of his suggestions.[422]

And, lastly, I want to draw your attention to work done in the field of psychohistory. Many papers have been published examining the connection of social violence such as war, violence against groups or individuals, and crime as an unconscious reenactment of prenatal trauma, the trauma of a violent birth, and abusive child-rearing practices. Findings in this field confirm that cultures that advocate gentle birth practices and nurturing models of child rearing often experience a significant reduction of social violence in all forms. See the note for suggested reading on this topic.[423]

Economic Stressors

The next wave of debilitating stress to affect a great number of people is economic stress. Let's use a specific example: the crisis of debt and foreclosure. This is a situation that in the last decade or so has been affecting more and more families and individuals in middle- and working-class America—the same sector of the population experiencing drastic rises in opioid deaths. The sustained mental and emotional stress commonly experienced during the months or years of economic worries, bankruptcy, or a foreclosure process is nothing less than toxic. This type of stress has been shown to increase the risk of developing chronic physical health issues (hypertension, diabetes, heart disease), mental-emotional problems (anxiety and depression), as well as increase opioid drug abuse.[424] But we are getting ahead of ourselves in predicting the outcome of an all-too-common story.

You buy a house, your slice of the American dream. You move in and make it your very own beautiful castle. It gives you and your loved ones shelter, warmth, a sense of safety, security, a place to be together and belong, among the many other tangible and intangible qualities that make life easier and worthwhile. Then something happens—a serious illness in the family, a loss of income, a layoff, or an economy going down the drain. You are struggling to make ends meet. You tread water and dig deeper into debt to keep afloat. Your debt is beginning to take its toll, getting worse until it feels like you are drowning. You take out a second loan to pay off the rising credit card bills. Now you are under water. You can't make your mortgage payments. The bank does not care. It has no heart; it is not human (no matter what Citizens United says) and exists solely to make more money, no matter what.

Economic insecurities and poverty have been determined to be major vulnerabilities for addiction. For instance, heroin addiction rates among people who have an annual income below $20,000 are more than three times higher than among people who make over $50,000.[425]

Faceless debt collectors with made-up names start calling. Bullying tactics intimidate with fear and instill guilt to force you to pay. If only you could. The emotional toll adds up. The shame and the stress from the constant bombardment and the hopelessness with no apparent solution in sight is not just unhealthy to your body and your mind, it can destroy families, crush your spirit, and tear away at your soul. Fear, anger, despair, and a slew of other debilitating emotions associated with bankruptcy or foreclosure often are unexpressed or inappropriately expressed. The constant contribution of these emotions exacerbates an already overwhelming experience of slowly losing your home and investment.

This scenario includes other vulnerabilities to addiction that together can produce the perfect storm: fear of survival, hopelessness, perceived loss of power to take care of yourself and your family, and silent or not so silent rage all chip away at your physical and emotional resilience. You may remember the example used in chapter 2 of an early study that correlated the social stress and increase of opioid use disorders (including overdose deaths) disproportionally experienced by communities subject to extreme austerity and economic stressors such as bankruptcy or foreclosure.[426] The abundance of addiction around the globe is a consequence of the mental-emotional pain caused when people are separated not only from meaningful work or adequate pay but also from cohesive traditional culture, nature, family, or spirituality. This includes the expectation or loss of the American dream, without doubt one of the major contributors to the current opioid epidemic in the United States.

Feeling Victim to Constricting Emotions: Lack of Emotional Self-Regulation Skill

In the previous chapter we highlighted specific neurotransmitter profiles and their emotional associates that are affected by the physical-emotional stress of opioid withdrawal. Approaches were suggested from mind-body medicine to regain and reestablish a more balanced profile. In addition, we can resolve that we will not be imprisoned by our emotions and can take steps to set ourselves free.

How might we begin the process of mapping out potential ways to rein in these emotions, develop more resilience, and thus be fortified in addressing personal crisis constructively? One way is to look for models and advice from people who have managed not just to survive but to thrive in the face of severe and constant stress from oppression that ruthlessly engenders challenging or overwhelming emotional experiences.

For instance, how did black South Africans handle the constant barrage of institutionalized racism rained upon them by the Apartheid system? After the fall of Apartheid, South Africans created a Truth and Reconciliation Committee that heard from perpetrators and their victims alike to begin the process of transparency and forgiveness as a way to heal the fear, anger, and hurt and to create opportunities to move on. Journalist Bill Moyers asked Desmond Tutu, one of the foremost leaders against Apartheid, "What do you actually do when you forgive someone?" Tutu responded, "Well, basically you're saying, 'I am abandoning my right to revenge, to payback.'"[427]

It would be difficult to find a culture or a spiritual belief system that does not praise the healing balm of forgiveness. We are told that every bit of forgiveness is a gift to you, not the other. Even modern science chimes in. A recent study conducted at the Department of Psychology at the University of Miami discovered that merely imagining forgiving someone else had a measurable effect on one's own health.[428] So why don't we do it more often?

Forgiveness is often mistaken for a weakness rather than seen as a strength. Some consider it a shortcut or a cop-out. Others believe forgiveness is a cheap justification to just do whatever you want. It is sometimes incorrectly characterized as giving up or admitting failure. Many people actually fear forgiveness, thinking that if they do forgive, they will reopen a wound, a hurt, a humiliation, and they don't want to ever deal with that "awful" feeling again. Or one might feel like forgiveness is saying that what another person did is OK when it wasn't. Others think forgiveness is arrogant, or "only God forgives." With beliefs like these, it is no wonder many don't try to engage the power contained in forgiveness.

To access the power in forgiveness it is essential to engage your capacity for thinking and feeling. Acknowledge whatever small or large part you may have played in allowing the bankruptcy or foreclosure (continuing our earlier example) to enter your experience. Think of it this way: "You can't sell the car unless you own it." Always take the first step on the road to forgiveness by forgiving yourself. Perhaps it is for a bad choice you made. Perhaps you will forgive yourself for the imprisoning fear or debilitating pain. Maybe the task is forgiving yourself for your ill-advised commitment to independence that refuses to let anybody help you. What can you learn from this situation? How do you feel about forgiving yourself? What resistances do you encounter? Can you forgive that resistance?

To own the car so you can sell it, to continue the analogy, try the following. In the privacy of a meditation, be with whatever feelings your responsibility engenders. Accept, embrace, and forgive that part of yourself. Now that you are forgiving yourself, consider what you don't have to do anymore. For instance, perhaps you can stop being so paranoid, stop being weak, stop being angry over and over again, or stop being ready to argue or fight at the drop of a hat. How does that feel?

As another powerful example, the people of Tibet continue to weather the omnipresent, violent oppression by the Chinese governmental forces with the directive to diminish the power, culture, and spiritual tradition of an entire people. In addition to forgiveness, the Dalai Lama, Tibet's spiritual leader, offers the way of compassion to subdue fear and despair. He applies reason, patience, and a compassionate attitude as an antidote to these imprisoning emotions: "If you have fear of some pain or suffering, you should examine whether there is anything you can do about it. If you can, there is no need to worry about it; if you cannot do anything, then there is also no need to worry."[429]

Considering compassion for yourself having to fight a hostile bank or aggressive debt collectors can be another nurturing and supportive power in your corner. Ask yourself: is getting angry with the bankers helping you hold onto your home? Is anger helping you to think things through with attention to the details? Is the constant presence of anger healthy for your body and your mind? Is losing your patience helping your sense of security and safety? Chances are the answers are no. This does not mean that you can't express yourself appropriately and employ strong countermeasures in return. Ask yourself if it is healthy to have compassion for yourself. Is it useful to step back and look at the bigger picture? Is it helpful to look at this crisis as a teacher from which you may learn something extraordinary? Chances are the answers could be yes.

The Dalai Lama offers a technique called Tong-Len (meaning giving and receiving) to strengthen the power of compassion within you. Tong-Len reverses the habit of avoiding suffering and seeking pleasure. Instead you seek out the disturbing thought. You visualize, in the safety of your mind, a group of people on one side of the room. Now, see these people suffering from turmoil and tragedy of all sorts such as homelessness, war, or loss of health or home. On the other side of the room imagine yourself as self-centered and indifferent to their suffering and pain. Now, in between that selfish you and the group of people in distress, place another representation of yourself as a neutral observer. Notice where you feel yourself naturally drawn. Looking objectively, chances are you will feel drawn to the group of people suffering. Now, metaphorically and energetically, take in all the suffering of that group of despondent people and give back love, joy, success, and any type of healing or soothing energy you can muster.

When we think we cannot do the meditation it is because we often come up against our own fears, anger, and despair. Now we can turn the practice on ourselves. Take in any present or imagined future suffering, such as your fear, anger, or despair, and send compassion and forgiveness to yourself. This is the core of Tong-Len.

In the depth of despair, both South Africans and Tibetans discovered a determined vision and commitment to bring about positive changes in non-violent ways. Both refuse being made to feel worthless by an all-powerful aggressor by reaching for something larger than any of them, such as a belief in some higher purpose, a deeper meaning, or a connection with something deeper or something spiritual or revered, defined by one's very personal experience or by the religious denomination of their choice.

What all three—forgiveness, compassion, and reaching for something larger than yourself—have in common is that they are subject to conscious intervention. Each is self-empowering and able to profoundly transform a life for the better. The more you recognize, take responsibility for (when necessary), and transcend your imprisoning emotions, and the more you strengthen your expansive ones, the more you shore up any possible vulnerability to addiction.

Other Vulnerabilities to Addiction and What Drives Them

Solely relying on a **policing** or a law-and-order approach reinforces vulnerabilities to addictions. The War on Drugs was based on the assumption that if drug availability is eliminated by prohibition, then addiction will cease to be a problem. We now know this hypothesis is false. In fact, it can be argued that prohibition of anything has rarely if ever worked. It didn't work in paradise. It doesn't work in jails or prisons. I have been called countless times to respond to police station holding cells and the city jail to treat patients who overdosed. If we can't keep drugs out of the most controlled environments in society, how is it going to work in open and free environments?

Consider the fallacy of the War on Drugs in comparison to the success of Portugal's nurturing approach to drugs and addiction,[430] mirrored in the recent finding indicating that states that allow for medicinal cannabis saw a 25 percent drop in opioid deaths.[431] Today, Portugal has one of the lowest numbers of drug-related deaths.[432] Despite having similar economic problems as Scotland, with one of the highest overdose death rates, Portugal differed in preventing a widespread erosion of hope by, instead of preaching abstinence and prohibition; instead of using law enforcement as a response to addiction; instead of cutting funds to prevention, treatment, and harm reduction measures, doing the opposite. Sixteen years later, solid evidence shows that the shift has paid off.

In 2001 Portugal demonstrated exceptional courage by going against the grain of global trends, against the negative predictions by "experts," and in the face of significant criticism from the majority of EU nations in dealing with drugs and addictions. Instead of viewing it as a criminal issue, it was now a public health issue. Possession of small amounts of all drugs was decriminalized, and Portugal created a holistic, multidisciplinary approach involving measures to reduce alienation and lack of meaning and create meaningful connection within society. In addition to free public health care for everyone, it created integrated health and social services for dealing with underlying trauma, pain, and mental health issues commonly associated with drug use and addiction. In addition to one of the lowest overdose deaths rate in Europe, HIV infection rates have dropped continuously since 2001, and thousands of former addicts have reentered and reconnected with society in meaningful and productive ways. Health care expenditures and societal costs savings are significant. Now the world is paying attention. Portugal is described as a glowing example of best possible practices to be copied or emulated.

The reader is advised that with all these positive changes implemented in Portugal, drugs larger than a ten-day supply of any substance are still illegal. High-volume drug dealing and trafficking is still a criminal offense, and violators are still incarcerated for more serious offenses. Those caught with small amounts will receive a ticket and must appear not before a court of law but a panel consisting of mental health, social, and legal professionals. The case is heard, and a unique response, consisting of hand-on practical steps, is prescribed, initiated, and set in motion to assure positive and sustainable results.

Relapse and Addiction Triggers

Common opioid use triggers or relapse triggers include: temptation by current opioid-using friends and places of use; quick and sudden changes (positive or negative); falling for heroin chic; the drama of a toxic romantic relationship; loneliness (not solitude), alienation, and disconnect; arrogance, hubris, or feeling overconfident; intolerable emotions and thoughts such as those generated by negative self-talk; consider the acronym HALT—hungry, angry, lonely, and tired.

Here is an interesting paradox. Using cannabis, like any behavior used to avoid an uncomfortable, painful, or otherwise difficult present moment, can become an unhealthy psychological habit, such as shopping, sex, exercise, and using alcohol and drugs. However, with the proper chemotype of cannabis for your particular situation and with conscious intention, it can also function to transcend any unhealthy habit. Many cannabis-using patients have reported that the deep relaxation associated with cannabis made it easier to discover their own trigger without judgment, and to relax in the presence of otherwise intolerable emotions and become aware of the reward dimensions. By looking at these things, we can gain impulse awareness and a better understanding of the value of our rewards, and thus be open to the possibility of new choices and options that replace any negative behaviors in the reaction phase with those that support our health and well-being.

Resistance to Healing Addiction

Another vulnerability presents itself when resistance to healing is present. This occurs when a part of the self attributes something positive to the presence of the disease. You may have heard the phrase, "It is very difficult to convince someone of the truth if their livelihood depends on not knowing it." In the context of addiction, perhaps the most challenging thing to do in deep healing is to examine the reasons why we might not want to heal. A reluctance to completely heal could be a reflection of our yearning for attention from others or a negative belief that stipulates we deserve this as punishment. Sometimes it might be misplaced family loyalties or the notion that "as long as I am sick he will never leave me." Perhaps addiction has become an identity or a way of life, an unhealthy way to get our needs met, or a means to feel special or in control. Perhaps we see our addiction as a way to avoid something, such as unwanted responsibilities, difficult emotions, or the judgment of others.

If this reluctance to give up on addiction as a hidden, secret means to whatever end is not addressed and resolved, one might consciously or unconsciously nourish the use disorder rather than oneself. Owning, forgiving, and releasing the resistance speeds recovery. Both the intentional use of cannabinoids and a mind-body approach can help to make it easier to learn about and be in the presence of our reluctances to healing. Here too, Tutu's and the Dalai Lama's suggestion of compassion and forgiveness *for oneself* can be great allies as we do our work with our shadow.

Managing Chronic Pain as an Isolated Physical Symptom

The reader is reminded that such a narrow approach is a limited view with potentially serious consequences. In fact, this omission of the greater context for opioid use constitutes another significant vulnerability for addiction. While opioids or cannabinoids can make a significant difference in pain management, ultimately neither one nor even both together can relieve all pain in the presence of a maintaining cause, such as unresolved or suppressed mental-emotional pain, continued unhealthy choices (cigarettes or food that's bad for you, an ongoing abusive relationship), or resistance to healing (seeing a benefit in the illness). Learning how to be resilient in the face of pain, and learning how to process all aspects of pain, including contributing causes, requires conscious participation and a sustained effort until the demand for change at the heart of pain is answered. That does not mean that we have to do it all alone. In fact, a healing team approach with the patient playing a strong participatory role is a model already proven to work.

Already mentioned in chapter 1 but worth repeating in the context of this discussion is that the 1980s saw the development of a multidisciplinary approach to healing chronic pain that included staff from various healing practices in one location, such as a physician, a physical therapist, and a psychologist. The healing team held regular meetings and discussed each patient's issues and progress. The team members assessed and treated the patients using a variety of comprehensive methodologies to work in concert, including a basic minimum of a physical exam, pharmaceutical management as needed, biopsychological evaluations, cognitive behavioral treatments for chronic pains, physical therapies, occupational therapies, and referrals to special care not in-house. A multidisciplinary approach (even at long-term follow-up) has been shown to significantly improve overall functioning, at lower cost, with an increased number of patients returning to work.[433]

Lack of Meaningful Connection

The loss of meaningful connection (such as social isolation) is an underlying circumstance contributing to vulnerability to substance abuse, and it is commonly found in people dealing with opioid use disorders or addictions. This contributing factor has been explored in great depth by Professor Emeritus Bruce K. Alexander, who has taught psychology and conducted addiction research in Vancouver, Canada, since the 1970s.[434]

Alexander was the first to posit, test, and prove that drugs are only a small part of the reality of addiction. This significant find stands in direct opposition to the narrative of the War on Drugs that was built on the notion that drugs are the sole cause of addiction and as such must be eradicated at all costs. This belief and approach are still at the basis of most global efforts to manage drugs and addiction. The now famous rat park experiments simply showed that mice chose to self-medicate with significant amounts of opioids when kept in tiny, isolated metal cages. When kept in a rat park[435] colony, however, with plenty of friends to socialize and mate with, and things to explore and play with, those rats rarely preferred opioids over water. The notion that drugs are the sole cause of addiction has also been upended by researchers who now recognize that sex, gambling, and internet addictions, among other obsessions, are engaging the same neurochemical mechanisms and neurological circuitry as that of addictive drugs.

Alexander went on to apply his observation from the rat park to the context of human addiction. In his dislocation theory of addiction, he posits that the spread of addiction on a globalizing planet can be linked more widely to unchecked free-market philosophies that can be imposed by any type of political power from the far left to the far right. Global capitalism produces an ever-growing gap between the haves and have-nots. As the middle class shrinks in the developed nations, more people perceive themselves among the have-nots. Most of the rest of the world is already in that camp. People are forced to relentlessly compete, work, and earn more in a so-called "race to the bottom," causing increased alienation and separation.[436] When the social belonging aspect of cohesive traditional tribal culture is ridiculed, denigrated, or destroyed by relocation, forced separation of families, or legal means, drug use and vulnerability to opioid addiction increase.[437]

Thus Alexander concludes that none of the current consensus approaches of law enforcement, prevention, and even treatment or harm prevention, will ultimately transcend the social phenomenon of addiction. Instead what's needed is a reboot of deeply held beliefs in capitalist principles that function with the cold brutality of a dog-eat-dog world to one that places tempering principles that benefit humans and the natural environment at least on par with the goal of maximizing profit. A good example is the emergence of human benefit corporations that take a balanced view of weighing both the heart and the purse, and endeavor to create public value with their business enterprise. Efforts to eliminate poverty, to acknowledge and rectify social injustices, to end harmful emissions, and to reduce unemployment are all part of the long game to end addiction.

Another voice constructively reframing the public view on drugs and addictions is that of Johan Hari,[438] who writes in great detail about the fallacies of the narrative of the War on Drugs and insightfully concludes that "the opposite of addiction is not sobriety; the opposite of addiction is connection."[439]

Shoring Up One's Defenses

In addition to the techniques already mentioned, here are a couple other approaches you might find useful.

Nature

A traditional and time-tested source of soothing and healing emotional pain is being in a beautiful natural setting. Despite the constant search for contemporary connection on social media, the **lack of connection with nature** has never been more apparent in human society. While jet-setting tourists share and "like" multiple images of cultural attractions, which constitute an ever-changing visual tapestry, few have learned to notice the seasonal pattern of the wind outside their window as it shifts throughout the seasons. Few have taken the time to appreciate the caterpillar transforming into the chrysalis and then the butterfly on the fennel weeds in their backyards. Few would be able to name the types of migratory birds living in the nature park just beyond the hill.

Connecting with nature is among the easiest and most accessible (for most people) activities to release stress and take in healing qualities of fresh air, beauty, awe, wonder, connection, and wholeness. It is a human grace that comes as easily as flight to an eagle. With every breath we inhale a gift given freely by the trees and plants. Our lungs take in oxygen and attach its molecules to the hemoglobin molecules in our red blood cells. We exhale the resulting carbon dioxide back into the atmosphere for the trees, plants, and algae to absorb for their nourishment and sustenance. With each breath we are intricately linked to the natural world. The simple act of breathing partakes in an elemental cycle of life—the atmospheric cycle of which we are an integral part.

That's why so many meditation practices focus on the breath. This focus connects us to ourselves, the air, and the moment. All one needs to realize a meaningful relationship with nature is an appreciation and understanding of these simplest of things we must do from moment to moment to exist. Breathe. Connect. Feel.

If you prefer working with the elements, consider a moving meditation. Find a quite space. Take your shoes off. Walk very slowly and intentionally. When you lift your foot, feel the lightness of space (air). When you move your foot forward, sense the warmth (fire) in your gliding joints. When you place your foot once again onto the ground, feel your connection with the earth. As the circle of movement begins again, become aware of the fluidity (water) of your motion.

Mindfulness

In many ways the word *mindfulness* has become a cliché, in the sense that you hear it everywhere, like elevator music, and as such it has lost much of its meaning and clarity. Some people tend to liken it to meditation or stress-reduction, while those on the other end of a definition spectrum tend to roll their eyes at the mere mention, thinking rose-colored glasses and Pollyanna.

However, in the context of this book, I am thinking of mindfulness in a clinical way that is rather precise. With a little practice people begin to witness their thoughts and feelings, not just when there are meditating but throughout the day, and their emerging impulses to act, without doing anything about it. So, when a trigger shows up that normally compels you to "use," you're in a better position to discern whether you want to act on it. It doesn't guarantee success, but it kind of puts the clutch on the engine when normally you'd be in drive already.

There are a great many mindfulness techniques, breathing practices, and meditations available for you to choose from. Allow me to share one that I personally use. About thirty years ago I was interested in learning about Buddhist philosophy and healing practices, and I went straight to the source. I traveled to Northern Thailand, to a town called Chiang Mai. Believing in learning by doing, I ordained as a monk. I lived at Wat Tapotaram, where the old Abbott taught me how to meditate using my breath. Kneeling on a meditation bench (I could never sit cross-legged for long), I listened intently as he taught me to focus my attention on my abdomen, about an inch or so above my navel, to place my mind's attention there. The focus point should lie on the vertical midline of the body.

As I breathe in, my abdomen expands until it peaks or pauses; as I breathe out, it contracts until I reach the bottom of the exhale or pause again. The monk said, "This never changes as long as you live." I found this thought oddly compelling and reassuring. As the abdomen expands, pauses, contracts, and pauses, follow the motion from beginning to end with your mind's eye. Just be with your breath throughout these four phases. That's all there is to it.

If you get distracted or your mind starts to wander, bring it gently back to that focus point on your belly. After I had some time to practice, I began to notice changes in my ability to maintain equanimity, and I experienced a deeper sense of peace and overall calm even when faced with a stressful situation. For many people, a meditation practice is an important resource to effectively manage a stress trigger or a chronically debilitating emotional state.

Researchers in the Department of Psychology at the University of Washington showed that mindfulness-based relapse prevention (MBRP) in substance use disorder demonstrates substantial efficacy as a therapy for addictive behaviors.[440] If you don't like to sit still but would like to practice meditation, you can look at moving meditations such as simple walking meditation mentioned earlier, tai chi, or qi gong, for example.

eight

The Pathologization of Euphoria: Rethinking the Idea that Euphoria Is a Side Effect and Reclaiming Its Capacity for Deep Healing

THE WORD *EUPHORIA* IS a compilation of the Greek words *eu,* meaning "good" or "well," and *pherō,* meaning "to bring" or "to bear." Euphoria is the opposite of dysphoria, where the bearer of good becomes the bearer of *dus,* "difficult," representing the constant state of unease.

Euphoria is commonly listed as an adverse side effect of both prescription opioids[441] and cannabinoids.[442] But what is so bad about having feelings of intense happiness, pleasure, and well-being? What is wrong with blissful elation, full-bodied gratitude, a euphoria so deep that all that remains is to wail with tears of joy? What is this force that inspires poets but seems to scare the institutions of government, to threaten the halls of modern medicine, and to attract suspicion in many organized houses of worship?

Medieval religious prejudices viewed ecstasy in two ways. Euphoria in the form of fun or of a voluptuous nature was considered a sign of the devil or demonic possession, especially in women. On the other hand, an extraordinary perception of a more immaculate nature was thought to be a vision from God—for example, the euphoric visions of Bernadette Soubirous led to her canonization and the establishment of the Sanctuary of Our Lady of Lourdes, France.

The limited response to the experience of euphoria was mirrored in the emerging orthodox medical profession of the eighteenth and nineteenth centuries. Medical professionals viewed both euphoria and its negative state, "possession," as a disease of the nervous system, and women afflicted with "the condition" were diagnosed with "hysteria," a term based on the Greek word *hustérā,* for "womb" or "uterus."

Let's think about it for a moment. Why is an emotional experience that otherwise could be described as a peak experience, an extraordinary state of consciousness, a heightened awareness, a moment of bliss, a sense of majesty, a brush with spirit, a touch of soul rich with substance, or an awareness of the immortal in oneself somehow thought to be an adverse effect like a skin rash or nausea? This judgment is even more irrational when we consider that expansive experiences of this nature can quickly shift neurological and psychological pain and dysphoria responses toward those that elicit expansive affect, which is clearly associated with therapeutic potential. You don't need to be a doctor to notice that this feels a heck of a lot better than depression or fear.

At about twenty years of age I had my first experience of euphoria. I had been drafted into the German Army and was stationed in Münster in North Rhine–Westphalia. One moment I had been a happy university student, and the next I was a rocket-artillery soldier and miserable as can be. The euphoric experience happened right after a medical procedure that required full anesthesia. When I came to, my parents were sitting next to my hospital bed with some mild concern on their faces. I lifted the blanket and looked at the stitches and severe swelling that had formed around the fresh incision shortly after the surgery was completed. But instead of concern, pain, or any discomfort, I was feeling a bliss like I never had before. I was flooded with love and joy. I felt a substantial amount of gratitude oozing out of every pore of my being.

I looked at my parents and told them I loved them. I don't remember ever saying it until that moment. It wasn't part of my upbringing to be demonstrative with affection or love. I could tell that while it was a little awkward for them, they liked it, as evidenced by their moist eyes. I don't remember how long it lasted, but it was my first euphoria—opioid-induced, but euphoria nevertheless. I loved it. I remember it clearly, brightly, and very fondly.

As the days of recovery progressed, the drugs were reduced, and I healed quickly. I was released from the hospital, and the moment of unconditional love shared with my parents was never mentioned again. At the time I had no idea how to integrate a peak experience into my relationships or my life in general. However, in hindsight I believe a seed was planted.

My second experience with euphoria was of a very different nature. Shortly after my conscription ended, I traveled to the United States for the first time. We were visiting a distant relative in Los Angeles. It didn't take long for me to be offered my first cannabis joint. (The reader is reminded that this was the eighties, when most cannabis was less than 5 percent THC content, and as such a fraction of what is commonly produced nowadays.) I inhaled a couple of times, and within minutes I started to break out laughing with spontaneous mirth. Laughter, and I mean a full belly type of laughter, exploded out of me nearly uncontrollably. Not that I wanted to control it. The cannabis-induced euphoria of mirth lasted about forty-five minutes, after which my belly ached a little, but I felt awash in the aftereffects: relaxed, gently energized, and right as rain.

A final euphoric experience I want to share (for reasons that will soon become clear) was initiated by yet another means. A woman friend of mine named Hanne, who was a naturopath ("Heilpraktiker") in Heilbronn, Germany, invited me to do a guided meditation just to see how I might like it. It was a simple technique that provided enough relaxation to create an altered state of consciousness, where the mind was let loose to explore itself using nothing but imagination, creativity, and the capacity for wonder.

At first it was nice and relaxing, but soon it became an intense, dreamlike journey, extremely vivid in its visual details. Hanne would occasionally check in with me, and I would respond by sharing a bit of my experience as it unfolded. After a while it became a gentle interaction. For example, I would describe standing in front of an abyss not knowing what to do. Hanne suggested asking for help to cross. As soon as I did, help arrived in the form of a tightrope spanning the entire gap. I was eased across with the help of an Indian deity and using a cross-bar for balance. Nothing seemed weird, just like nothing is ever logical in a dream. On the other side, an inner adventure began that culminated in a sense of majesty, a moment in time that revealed a bit of the immortal. I eventually emerged from the journey in tears, having been touched emotionally and spiritually in ways I had never been touched before.

To this day I practice a form of guided meditation to replenish myself when feeling depleted, to get inspiration when lacking direction, to connect when feeling lost, and, of course, to ask for help when faced with challenges, obstacles, or seemingly insurmountable odds. These three forms of euphoria were produced by different means: opioids, cannabinoids, and a mindfulness technique. Each of these temporary moments of bliss was part of a healing I needed at the time, and they still inform me, assist me, and resonate within me as a resource to this day.

Euphoria is one of the most underrated, underutilized, and prosecuted forces of healing, transformation, and transcendence known to humankind. Seeking euphoria is an intrinsic behavior of humanity. It is a behavioral constant. Meanwhile it is bias, prejudice, and moral judgment that serve to frame the pleasure of euphoric bliss as a pathology.

In fact, it's not just people who seek out euphoria. Siberian reindeer and North American caribou actively seek out fly agaric mushrooms *(Amanita muscaria),* the legendary red mushroom with white dots, and feed on them abundantly until the animals become severely altered in their behavior. They make unusual noises and slowly move their rear ends, their snouts begin to twitch, and they wander about with swaying steps.

Overripe fermenting durian fruit are a favorite of elephants and monkeys, who eat as much as they can until they are too drunk, at which point they lie down or move in slow motion. When the effects wear off, they go straight back for more until the supply is exhausted. The same is true for certain birds in the United States. When cherries become ripe and begin to ferment on the tree, birds of all types flock to the feast and gorge themselves until they fall to the ground. If left alone, they return for more as soon as their faculties allow them to.

When was the last time you experienced something so beautiful it moved you to tears? When was the last time you had a cascading orgasm of joy?

The thrill of a profound spiritual experience? A feeling of deep connection with all that is without losing your sense of individuality? Did you ever have a breakthrough, a sudden insight, a palpable touch of truth brush up against your essence? Many of us do. For some it is a life-changing event with real practical and measurable consequences, while for others it became a fond but fading memory and lost opportunity (at least for now). What can be done to nourish the seedling of transcendent potential at the core of a euphoric moment? How do we increase the chances of integrating an experience of bliss into one that becomes a steady ally or a constant resource in our ongoing quest for deeper healing and evolution?

Deconstructing the sensory details of a euphoric experience similar to the process used in method acting,[443] for instance, can function as a useful strategy in taking agency by first recalling the experience the way it felt to you in your body. And rather than following the understandable temptation of thinking about the burst of ideas, visions, and dreams, consider for starters just staying with sensing if or how your body feels different in or since this euphoric shift. You might find it a completely new experience, such as a new sense of aliveness or vitality. It may show up as a feeling (a buzz, vibration, or sound). Just note the subtle feeling differences. Some people might find the newness disconcerting. If that is the case, notice that as well.

Next you may want to consider how you feel about these sensations. Notice what thoughts arise—the quality of your self-talk, for example. Are you telling yourself, "That was nice, but it won't last?" And if so, do you want to run with that? Do you want to believe that? If not, what belief would you rather hold? Remember, those thoughts, those emotions, those choices we repeat over and over become the path of least resistance. Those become the hardwired response that determines our experiences. Try to build pathways that give you a sense of wonder, curiosity, support, safety, or other nurturing qualities, and you will in turn shift and change your chemistry into those of the same qualities.

While the forces of prohibition, the policies of fear and war and oppression, are still omnipresent in too many parts of the world, new possibilities are already emerging and making their real and substantial impact known.

There is a Native American prayer we can remember in times of need: "I give thanks for help already on the way."

Long-held attitudes are slowly but surely being tempered and replaced by informed discernment as science-based explorations continue to advance and recognize the therapeutic potential and benefits of the extraordinary states of consciousness induced by substances such as opioids (for cancer patients with intractable pain, for example), cannabis (for AIDS wasting syndrome),[444] ecstasy (in the treatment of PTSD),[445] psilocybin mushrooms[446] and LSD[447] (for easing anxiety when dying), as well as *Tabernanthe iboga* (in the treatment of severe heroin addiction).[448] Euphoria isn't just a breakthrough high; it can be breakthrough therapy, healing, and lasting change. Euphoria and other altered states of consciousness, peak experiences, extraordinary states of awareness, or whatever name one gives these experiences are beginning to reclaim their value in healing specific health concerns such as chronic pain, in transcending the human condition in addiction, and in shifting the societal resonance to looking inward for growth and resolution.

nine

Conclusion: Putting It All Together

IN VIEW OF THE current epidemic of opioid-based overdoses and deaths, it should be widely proclaimed, first and foremost, that supplementing chronic pain management with cannabis is a proven avenue to implementing a number of harm-reduction factors. These include realizing the effective analgesia of opioids but at lower dosages, reducing the risk of adverse effects, and cutting back on the tragic incidence of fatal overdoses. Then there is the factor of individual savings to the wallet and the overburdened health care system. An opioid habit can cost around a $100 a day, while supplementing with about 1 gram of cannabis flower (which is often more than enough) costs about $10 to $15. If taking the two synergistically, the quantity of opioid can be reduced to get the same effects—which are delivered along with the myriad other benefits of cannabinoids in one's regimen.

Endogenous (meaning the body's own) cannabinoids and opioids are natural and essential to how the human body and mind heal. When we are balanced, healthy, and resilient, they are extremely capable systems to handle the temporary challenges of an injury or emotional wound. However, in the presence of chronic stressors (maintaining causes, illness, pain, loneliness, substance withdrawal), the body's naturally occurring opioid and cannabinoid response systems can become both overwhelmed and imbalanced. In this case, the body can benefit from some help from their plant-based relatives. It is only natural that in the pursuit of health and healing, we learn to effectively and appropriately use the original plant-based versions of these therapeutic gifts of nature.

The aim of this book is to provide readers with some basic suggestions and discernment on how to use both as effectively and safely as possible. Here in the book's conclusion I'd like to review important highlights and to summarize some of the book's main points.

Anyone managing chronic pain must be aware that neither opioids nor cannabinoids, or their combination, is a silver bullet to magically relieve pain indefinitely. These medicines, powerful as they are, will never fully substitute for conscious involvement in the healing process, especially when pains and illnesses are chronic. For instance, neither will be able to change a maintaining cause of pain. Neither will be able to make healthier lifestyle and nutrition choices for you. While you may experience a shift in the internal architecture of the mind—and with it feel what it is like to be relaxed instead of tense, to be happy instead of hurt, or to feel love instead of fear—neither will be able to permanently replace an unhealthy belief with one that nurtures you. And while both plants may help you experience what it is like to feel good about yourself (a sense of feeling OK and belonging to the web of life, kindness toward self, or a tangible moment of self-love and self-appreciation), neither will sustain your positive self-image if you insist on feeding a negative one with your thoughts and statements.

Perhaps an opioid or cannabinoid high will flood you with a temporary sense of gratitude, forgiveness, or compassion and a desire to make necessary changes in your life, but if you ultimately cannot break unhealthy habits (poor foods, negative self-talk, guilt, excess stress), you will fall right back to walking the path of least resistance and doing the things that may have brought your health to the brink of collapse in the first place. Your old, narrow synaptic clefts will fire with cold precision set in motion by your habit of destructive mental constructs that are biologically implemented by corresponding negative neurotransmitter profiles.

As this book tries to convey throughout, both our biology and psychology are subject to conscious intervention, and this presents a key window of opportunity for healing. While it may take greater initial efforts to build new and more positive neuronal pathways, when the pathways and messages of chronic pain and chronic dysphoria (e.g., withdrawal) are overwhelmingly omnipresent, it is work worth doing to improve quality of life. Indeed, if deep healing, not just temporary relief, is your goal, the work to change mind and body internally becomes essential.

Let's review some critical points.

Opium poppies are unique plants that provide the natural basis for opiates, which, properly used, are well known to reduce pain and facilitate healing during acute episodes. But as we all know by now, opioids carry very real risks, especially when used for long periods of time, when used at higher concentrations than necessary, or when used inappropriately (a.k.a. abused).

Cannabis can temper these risks and thus support one's healing process in a number of ways, ranging from reducing the risk of opioid-based adverse effects to boosting its analgesic ability to setting the stage for realizing and replacing unhealthy habits or choices. The latter occurs by producing a subtle shift in consciousness. It is not a stretch to think of the conscious and intentional use of cannabis as a powerful mindfulness technique.

It is critical to remember (especially if you are new to using cannabis in any manner) that not all cannabis is the same. For instance, THC (psychoactive) and CBD (nonpsychoactive) produce a great number of unique effects and at the same time produce similar effects but by different means (see figure 3.2 in chapter 3). Therefore, the more you know about the therapeutic abilities of THC and CBD, the more empowered you will be to take charge of the type of cannabis-induced effects and experience you wish, or need, to have (see figure 3.1 in chapter 3).

One of the most meaningful and practical distinctions necessary to match your desired effect, in terms of symptom reduction or mood improvements, with the type of cannabis best suited to deliver this effect is the distinction among the three basic cannabis chemotypes.

Chemotype I contains more THC than CBD. **Chemotype II** contains relatively equal amounts of THC to CBD, close to 1:1. **Chemotype III** contains more CBD than THC, or no THC at all. This basic measure is true for cannabis flowers and any other cannabis-containing product.

For instance, in the case of needed analgesic effects, chemotype-based discernments can offer an up-to-date scientific basis to build and sustain informed choices about how to supplement your pain management with cannabinoids. The process requires a little or a lot of trial and error for most people, and this will be true until scientific research is free to fully study the potential of cannabis and develop truly targeted medicines. Chapter 4 offers a select evidence-based risk-versus-benefit analysis of what types of pains tend to respond well to opioids versus cannabinoids, and in which cases one or the other is more questionable and still subject to ongoing study and debate. Here is a summary:

Treating Central Pain (Neuropathies)

- **opioids:** poor–possible
- **cannabinoids:** possible (chemotype range I–III)

Treating Peripheral Pain (Neuropathies)

- **opioids:** poor
- **cannabinoids:** possible–good (chemotype range primarily II, with minor evidence for I)

Treating Acute Pain

- **opioids:** good
- **cannabinoids:** poor (chemotype range not applicable)

Treating Chronic Pain

- **opioids:** poor–possible
- **cannabinoids:** possible–good (chemotype range I–III)

Treating Nociceptive Pain

- **opioids:** good in acute self-limiting injuries, poor–possible in cases of chronic pain
- **cannabinoids:** possible (chemotype range I–II)

Treating Inflammatory Pain

- **opioids:** poor–possible
- **cannabinoids:** good (chemotype range I–III)

Treating Pathological Pain

- **opioids:** poor
- **cannabinoids:** possible–good (chemotype I)

Treating Mental-Emotional Suffering

- **opioids:** Makes you forget about it temporarily but does not change the cause.
- **cannabinoids:** Can set the stage for exploration and revelation. Can make intolerable emotions OK. May assist in resolution. (Chemotype range I–III)

Treating Opioid Withdrawal

- **opioids:** possible–good
- **cannabinoids:** possible–good (chemotype range I-III)

Understanding cannabis chemotypes is also relevant in cases of opioid withdrawal. Consider the notable trend for some patients with severe opioid withdrawal symptoms where the use of a highly concentrated version of THC (for example, dabbing with 90 percent THC) is preferred to achieve rapid relief; then over time, slowly moving toward using a flower of chemotype I with a high concentration of THC (>28 percent) to achieve similar effects but at lower concentrations. As neurotransmitter profiles are restored, patients may wish to continue to shift toward the chemotype III end of the spectrum (see Chapter 5)—the idea being that as you begin to heal by reestablishing the endocannabinoid-modulated balance of your organ systems, less external substance (lower THC percentage) are needed, and eventually your body can stand completely on its own versions of cannabinoids by having recreated a balanced state that is resilient in the face of life stressors (see chapter 7).

A balanced state and strong resilience can be built, rebuilt, and supported by participating in activities that shore up any potential vulnerabilities and support healthy, free-flowing neurotransmitter profiles. This is accompanied by a healthy and mindful mental and emotional response ability that comes from identifying and releasing unhealthy habits and replacing them with healthy ones.

One such habit is finding and cultivating positive means of creating healthy and natural euphoria-like moments and events. They may include close, vulnerable, intimate conversations with a trusted friend. Such moments and people in your life can be especially valuable when it comes to releasing a sorrow, a thing you did, a thing you regret, a thing you can't undo. It's the religious idea of confession—the notion in the twelve-step process where you take an inventory of specific wrongs committed and acknowledge the harm they caused and how it must have felt to the other person. Eventually one must come to terms with the past, not with self-loathing or self-punishment but with genuine empathy and sorrow—*even for oneself.* Make amends if appropriate. And when you are unsure how to proceed, consider applying the old Wiccan rede (moral code): "Do as thou will with harm to none." However, many people inflict the harm on themselves and not others. This tendency also must be acknowledged and uprooted.

A simple-appearing but mentally emotional complex process of this nature can be cathartic and produce connection, change, and euphoria. Others might find euphoria-like feelings in connecting with nature's beauty, or in the simple relationship with one of her most loving and accessible creatures—a dog, for example. A dear friend of mine told me about a time when she caught her dog just looking at her. In this moment she sensed that her dog was looking at her with an incredible abundance of love. She said she opened to really let it in, and it filled her with joy that overflowed in tears—her favorite kind of euphoria.

Other might feel more drawn to one of many mindfulness techniques. Still others might find it possible to cultivate euphoria by taking love-making to a deeper and more intimate experience. Orgasm certainly qualifies as a euphoric experience. But what if the entire sexual experience and not just the culmination could be elevated to euphoria? For those of you who find this avenue tempting, consider learning about tantra and its methods of heightening sensual and sexual energy, allowing it to go to a higher octave such that euphoria becomes a steady string of moments rather than just a single peak experience.

As you may have noticed, none of these ideas or practices cost anything but some time and energy spent to examine and come to terms with your past, or to learn something new. This is the point. Depending on intensity, chronic pain or chronic dysphoria are an invitation or demand for change. This brings us to another important consideration.

Dosage Considerations

Determining the proper dose of cannabis or a cannabis-containing product depends primarily on two factors: one, your individual need, preference, and tolerance; and two, what kind of product you choose. For instance, if you need quick and short-term relief, you may choose to inhale vaporized cannabis. If you need longer-term effects, you may want to work with an ingestible form.

To arrive at the most precise means and method to realize and sustain desired effects, it is helpful to determine the exact amount of THC. You might ask why only THC and not CBD? This is because THC is the psychotropic element of cannabis that can make the experience miserable for people when they get too much in their system—especially people who are new to these effects. If you're using tested products, the ratio between THC and CBD will be clearly marked, allowing you to know the exact value of THC, from which you'll be able to infer the exact value of CBD. For instance, if you are using a chemotype I with more THC than CBD at a ratio of 10:1, then you know that the amount of CBD will be one tenth that of THC (10:1).

For practical purposes, since only THC is psychoactive, it is generally advisable and easier to calculate precision values based on THC. Once you know THC-based effects based on milligrams, you will be able to adjust among different products and sustain desirable effects with only a few minor calculations. For some people, inhaling a total of 5 mg of THC is sufficient to produce their desired therapeutic effects, while others may need 300 mg to achieve efficacy. This dosage quantity is not to be confused with the weight of the flower, because THC content depends on percent concentration, which can vary greatly in a cannabis sample.

THC-ONLY DOSAGE CONSIDERATIONS (VIA INHALATION)

THC micro dose	~0.1 mg to 0.3 mg
THC low dose	~0.5 mg to 5 mg
THC medium dose	~6 mg to 20 mg
THC higher dose	~21 mg to 50+ mg

The reader is reminded that ingestible forms of THC require much less than the quantity typically inhaled (smoked or vaporized). Statistical analysis, echoed by experiences from cannabis-using patients, suggests an amount of THC for eating that is **six times less than inhaling.** For example, if you were satisfied with smoking 30 mg of THC, you'd need only 5 mg in an ingestible form to achieve the same results. Remember also that ingesting takes up to two hours, depending on stomach contents, to feel effects, so be patient. There is indeed a fine line between realizing therapeutic effects and shooting past your subjective therapeutic window and manifesting adverse effects.

Following are some sample dosage recommendations of pharmaceutical cannabinoid-based products, which roughly mirror average patient experiences using cannabis flower or cannabis-containing edibles.

Chemotype I: dronabinol (1:0) contains a synthetic version of THC and comes in dosages of 2.5 mg, 5 mg, and 10 mg soft gelatin capsules. Trials suggest effective dosage ranges between 2.5 mg and 20 mg.

Chemotype II: Sativex (1:1). Each spray contains 2.7 mg THC and 2.5 mg CBD. Patients are usually advised to titrate to effect and to stop if unwanted effects occur. Trials suggest effective dosage ranges between 5 and 10 sprays per day or 13.5 mg THC and 27 mg THC total per day.[449]

Chemotype III: Epidiolex (0:1) comes as an oral solution of plant-derived CBD only. A meta-analysis of trials conducted on pediatric patients suffering from treatment-resistant epilepsy indicated that patients were given amounts ranging between 10 mg/kg (which were considered efficacious and well tolerated) and 20 mg/kg per day.[450] Another review discovered that long-term use and high doses up to 1,500 mg per day of CBD were well tolerated in humans.[451]

Readers curious about common strain names of each chemotype may refer to Figure 3.3 in Chapter Three.

CBD-ONLY DOSAGE CONSIDERATIONS (VIA INGESTION)

CBD low dose	0.4 mg to 20 mg
CBD medium dose	20 mg to 100 mg
CBD high dose	100 mg to 800+ mg

Whether you're using opioids or cannabinoids or a combination of them, it can be argued that the quality of our emotions determines the quality of our lives. Using drugs (or any activity) that produces the way we want to feel is a form of emotional self-regulation. Ultimately, what our drug-taking reveals, by the emotions they engender, is what kind of emotional life we truly are looking for. In a way, our drug-taking demonstrates substantial aspects of our dreams, purpose, and meaning.

For the past two centuries, those who felt the call to "high" adventure flocked to San Francisco in the hopes of realizing the way they wanted to live, the way they wanted to feel. Similarly, we each have our own version of why we might be using a mind-altering substance. Many cannabis-using people seek relaxation, ease, and lightheartedness to cope with the ill effects of too much chronic stress or too much unresolved emotional pain. Many opioid-using people seek analgesic euphoria (to feel OK) in the face of seemingly never-ending physical pain, and many others are trying to ease pain of a mental-emotional nature. What is it for you? What kind of life do you want to live, and what kind of emotions would give it to you? A final question worth considering is, what is the most life-affirming way to realize it?

Take good care of yourself!

NOTES

1 Pamela T.M. Leung, Erin M. Macdonald, Irfan A. Dhalla, and David N. Juurlink, "A 1980 Letter on the Risk of Opioid Addiction," *New England Journal of Medicine* 376 (2017), 2194–95; R. K. Portenoy and K. M. Foley, "Chronic Use of Opioid Analgesics in Nonmalignant Pain: Report of 38 Cases," *Pain* 25:2 (May 1986), 171–86; San Francisco Medical Examiner's Office, *Annual Report, July 1, 1998–June 30, 1999,* 1999:65; K. H. Seal, A. H. Kral, L. Gee, et al., "Predictors and Prevention of Nonfatal Overdose Among Street-Recruited Injection Heroin Users in the San Francisco Bay Area, 1998–1999," *American Journal of Public Health* 91:11 (2001), 1842–46.

2 B. D. Sites, M. L. Beach, and M. Davis, "Increases in the Use of Prescription Opioid Analgesics and the Lack of Improvement in Disability Metrics Among Users," *Regional Anesthesia and Pain Medicine* 39:1 (2014), 6–12.

3 Ibid.

4 U.S. Centers for Disease Control and Prevention (CDC), "Provisional Counts of Overdose Deaths, as of August 6, 2017," www.cdc.gov/nchs/data/health_policy/monthly-drug-overdose-death-estimates.pdf.

5 Pradip K. Muhuri, Joseph C. Gfroerer, and M. Christine Davies, "Associations of Nonmedical Pain Reliever Use and Initiation of Heroin Use in the United States," *Center for Behavioral Health Statistics and Quality Data Review,* August 2013, http://goo.gl/T1ydQi.

6 Wilson M. Compton, Christopher M. Jones, and Grant T. Baldwin, "Relationship between Nonmedical Prescription-Opioid Use and Heroin Use," *New England Journal of Medicine* 374 (2016), 154–63.

7 G. A. Beauchamp, E. L. Winstanley, S. A. Ryan, and M. S. Lyons, "Moving Beyond Misuse and Diversion: The Urgent Need to Consider the Role of Iatrogenic Addiction in the Current Opioid Epidemic," *American Journal of Public Health* 104:11 (2014), 2023–29.

8 Ibid.

9 "Conversation with Raphael Mechoulam," *Addiction* 102 (2007), 887–93.

10 M. A. Bachhuber, B. Saloner, C. O. Cunningham, and C. L. Barry, "Medical Cannabis Laws and Opioid Analgesic Overdose Mortality in the United States, 1999–2010," *JAMA Internal Medicine* 174:10 (2014), 1668–73.

11 Amanda Reiman, Mark Welty, and Perry Solomon, "Cannabis as a Substitute for Opioid-Based Pain Medication: Patient Self-Report," *Cannabis and Cannabinoid Research* 2:1 (June 2017), 160-166.

12 C. E. Hughes and A. Stevens, "A Resounding Success or a Disastrous Failure: Reexamining the Interpretation of Evidence on the Portuguese Decriminalization of Illicit Drugs," *Drug and Alcohol Review* 31:1 (January 2012), 101–13.

13 C. B. Johannes, T. K. Le, X. Zhou, J. A. Johnston, and R. H. Dworkin, "The Prevalence of Chronic Pain in United States Adults: Results of an Internet-Based Survey," *Jounal of Pain* 11 (2010), 1230–39.

14 B. Levy, L. Paulozzi, K. A. Mack, and C. M. Jones, "Trends in Opioid Analgesic-Prescribing Rates by Specialty, U.S., 2007–2012," *American Journal of Preventive Medicine* 49:3 (September 2015), 409–13.

15 D. Manjiani, D. B. Paul, S. Kunnumpurath, A. D. Kaye, and N. Vadivelu, "Availability and Utilization of Opioids for Pain Management: Global Issues," *The Ochsner Journal* 14:2 (2014), 208–15.

16 R. Chou, R. Deyo, B. Devine, et al., *The Effectiveness and Risks of Long-Term Opioid Treatment of Chronic Pain* (Rockville, MD: Agency for Healthcare Research and Quality, 2014), www.ncbi.nlm.nih.gov/books/NBK258809.

17 Center for Behavioral Health Statistics and Quality, *2014 National Survey on Drug Use and Health: Detailed Tables* (Rockville, MD: Substance Abuse and Mental Health Services Administration, 2015).

18 Center for Behavioral Health Statistics and Quality, *Key Substance Use and Mental Health Indicators in the United States: Results from the 2015 National Survey on Drug Use and Health*, HHS Publication SMA 16-4984 (2016), 21.

19 Muhuri et al., "Associations of Nonmedical Pain Reliever Use."

20 Center for Behavioral Health Statistics and Quality, *Key Substance Use*, 21.

21 M. Noble, J. R. Treadwell, S. J. Tregear, V. H. Coates, P. J. Wiffen, C. Akafomo, K. M. Schoelles, and R. Chou, "Long-term Opioid Management for Chronic Noncancer Pain," *Cochrane Database of Systematic Reviews* 1 (CD006605:2010), doi:10.1002/14651858. CD006605.pub2; K. E. Vowles, M. L. McEntee, P. S. Julnes, T. Frohe, J. P. Ney, and D. N. van der Goes, "Rates of Opioid Misuse, Abuse, and Addiction in Chronic Pain: A Systematic Review and Data Synthesis," *Pain* 156:4 (April 2015), 569–76; Lee N. Robins, John E. Helzer, Michie Hesselbrock, and Eric Wish, "Three Years after Vietnam: How Our Study Changed Our View of Heroin," *The American Journal on Addictions* 19, 203–11.

22 William von Hippel, Loren Brener, and Courtney von Hippel, "Implicit Prejudice Toward Injecting Drug Users Predicts Intentions to Change Jobs Among Drug and Alcohol Nurses," *Psychological Science* 19:1 (January 2008), 7–11.

23 R. Room, "Stigma, Social Inequality, and Alcohol and Drug Use," *Drug and Alcohol Review* 24 (2005), 143–55.

24 Dan Werb, Thomas Kerr, Bohdan Nosyk, Steffanie Strathdee, Julio Montaner, and Evan Wood, "The Temporal Relationship between Drug Supply Indicators: An Audit of International Government Surveillance Systems," *BMJ Open* 3:9 (September 30, 2013).

25 National Center for Biotechnology Information, "PubChem Compound Database," CID=62156, http://pubchem.ncbi.nlm.nih.gov/compound/62156. Accessed September 9, 2017.

26 U.S. Drug Enforcement Agency (DEA), *Headquarters News,* September 22, 2016, www.dea .gov/divisions/hq/2016/hq092216.shtml.

27 U.S. CDC, "Provisional Counts of Overdose Deaths."

28 Long title: An Act to provide for the registration of, with collectors of internal revenue, and to impose a special tax upon all persons who produce, import, manufacture, compound, deal in, dispense, sell, distribute, or give away opium or coca leaves, their salts, derivatives, or preparations, and for other purposes. Short title: Harrison Narcotics Tax Act. Effective March 1, 1915.

29 Leung et al., "1980 Letter."

30 Ibid.

31 Barry Meier, "In Guilty Plea, OxyContin Maker to Pay $600 Million," *New York Times* Business Day, May 10, 2007, www.nytimes.com/2007/05/10/business/11drug-web.html.

32 Ravi Gupta, Nilay D. Shah, and Joseph S. Ross, "The Rising Price of Naloxone: Risks to Efforts to Stem Overdose Deaths," *New England Journal of Medicine* 375 (2016), 2213–15.

33 Ibid.

34 Physician Payments Sunshine Act of 2009, www.congress.gov/bill/111th-congress /senate-bill/301.

35 H. Flor, T. Fydrich, and D. C. Turk, "Efficacy of Multidisciplinary Pain Treatment Centers: A Meta-analytic Review," *Pain* 49 (1992), 221–30; A. H. Roberts, R. A. Sternbach, and J. Polich, "Behavioral Management of Chronic Pain and Excess Disability: Long-Term Follow-up of an Outpatient Program," *Clin. J. Pain* 9 (1993), 41–48; S. J. Kamper, A. T. Apeldoorn, A. Chiarotto, R. J. Smeets, R. W. Ostelo, J. Guzman, and M. W. van Tulder, "Multidisciplinary Biopsychosocial Rehabilitation for Chronic Low Back Pain: Cochrane Systematic Review and Meta-analysis," *BMJ* 350 (2015), h444; L. E. Patrick, E. M. Altmaier, and E. M. Found, "Long-Term Outcomes in Multidisciplinary Treatment of Chronic Low Back Pain: Results of a 13-Year Follow-up," *Spine* 29 (2004), 850–55.

36 H. Robbins, R. J. Gatchel, C. Noe, N. Gajraj, P. Polatin, M. Deschner, A. Vakharia, and L. Adams, "A Prospective One-Year Outcome Study of Interdisciplinary Chronic Pain Management: Compromising Its Efficacy by Managed Care Policies," *Anesthesia & Analgesia* 97 (2003), 156–62; R. J. Gatchel, C. E. Noe, N. M. Garaj, A. S. Vakharia, P. B. Polatin, M. Dreschner, and C. Pulliam, "Treatment carve-out practices: their effect on managing pain at an interdisciplinary pain center," *J. Work. Comp.* 10 (2001), 50–63.

37 J. N. Campbell, "APS 1995 Presidential address," *Pain Forum* 5 (1996) 85–8.

38 "The FDA Takes a Stand Against an Opioid that Fueled an Epidemic," *The Washington Post*, June 12, 2017.

39 C. Conrad, H. M. Bradley, D. Broz, et al., "Community Outbreak of HIV Infection Linked to Injection Drug Use of Oxymorphone, Indiana, 2015," *Morbidity and Mortality Weekly Report* 64:16 (2015), 443–4; S. A. Strathdee and C. Beyrer, "Threading the Needle—How to Stop the HIV Outbreak in Rural Indiana," *New England Journal of Medicine* 373:5 (2015), 397–9.

40 Food and Drug Administration, Office of the Commissioner, "Press Announcements: FDA Requests Removal of Opana ER for Risks Related to Abuse," www.fda.gov. Accessed June 15, 2017.

41 D. C. McDonald, K. Carlson, and D. Izrael, "Geographic Variation in Opioid Prescribing in the U.S.," *Journal of Pain* 13:10 (2012), 988–96.

42 U.S. Drug Enforcement Agency, Miami Division, "Miami News: Florida Doctors No Longer Among the Top Oxycodone Purchasers in the United States," April 5, 2013, www .dea.gov/divisions/mia/2013/mia040513.shtml.

43 Department of Justice, Office of Public Affairs, "AlphaBay, the Largest Online 'Dark Market,' Shut Down," July 20, 2017, www.justice.gov/opa/pr/alphabay-largest-online-dark-market -shut-down.

44 Nicander of Colophon, *Theriaca et Alexipharmaca* (Leipzig: B. G. Teubner, 1856), 433–64.

45 B. Trancas, N. Borja Santos, and L. D. Patrício, "The Use of Opium in Roman Society and the Dependence of Princeps Marcus Aurelius," *Acta Med Port* 21:6 (November-December 2008), 581–90.

46 Global Biodiversity Information Facility, GBIF Backbone Taxonomy, "*Papaver somniferum* L.," Sp. pl. 1:508. http://doi.org/10.15468/39omei. Accessed August 21, 2017.

47 D. I. Macht, "The History of Opium and Some of Its Preparation and Alkaloids," *JAMA* 64 (1915), 477–61.

48 P. G. Kritikos and S. P. Papadaki, "The History of the Poppy and of Opium and Their Expansion in Antiquity in the Eastern Mediterranean Area," United Nations Office on Drugs and Crime *Bulletin* 19:3 (1967), n. 126, www.unodc.org/unodc/en/data-and-analysis/bulletin /bulletin_1967-01-01_3_page004.html.

49 C. E. Terry, *The Opium Problem* (New York: Bureau of Social Hygiene, 1928), 54.

50 H. J. Anslinger and W. F. Tompkins, *The Traffic in Narcotics* (New York: Funk and Wagnalls, 1953), 1; Kritikos and Papadaki, "History of the Poppy."

51 Helen Askitopoulou, Ioanna A. Ramoutsaki, and Eleni Konsolaki, "Archaeological Evidence on the Use of Opium in the Minoan World," *International Congress Series* 1242 (December 2002), 23–29.

52 Ibid.

53 Saber Gabra, "Papaver Species and Opium through the Ages," *Bulletin de l'Institut d'Egypte* 1956, 40; H. R. Hall, "Notices of Recent Publications," *Journal of Egyptian Archaeology* 14 (1928).

54 Hesiod, *Theogony,* 11.535–37.

55 Johann Gottlob Schneider, *Orpheus' Argonautica,* 1803, 11.914–15.

56 *Iliad* 9.306–7; *Odyssey* 10.220–32.

57 Trancas et al., "Use of Opium in Roman Society."

58 A. Tschirch, *Handbuch der Pharmakognosie I/III,* 1933, 1208, 1209; Winifred Walker, *The Plants of the Bible* (London: Lutterworth, 1959), 88.

59 Jerusalemin Talmud, Tr. Abodah Zarah, 40a.

60 H. Askitopoulou, I. A. Ramoutsaki, and E. Konsolaki, "Analgesia and Anesthesia: The Etymology and Literary History of Related Greek Words," *Analgesia & Anesthesia* 91:2 (2000), 486–91.

61 Hippocrates, *Œuvres complètes d'Hippocrate,* On Epidemics 2.118; On Diet, chap. 39; On the Nature of Women, chap. 33; On Women's Ailments, chap. 20.

62 Aristotle, Physica Minora, 456b, 30; Historia Animalium I.6276, 18.

63 Claudii Galeni, *Medicorum Graecorum opera quae exstant* (Leipzig: B. G. Teubner, 1826), vol. XIII, 273.

64 Thomas Sydenham, *The Works of Thomas Sydenham,* trans. R. G. Latham (London: Sydenham Society, 1848), vol. I, xcix.

65 David Dary, *Frontier Medicine* (New York: Alfred Knopf, 2008), 36.

66 John M. Dorsey, ed., *The Jefferson-Dunglison Letters* (Charlottesville, VA: University of Virginia Press, 1960), 41–42.

67 Peter J. Hatch and Edwin Morris Betts, *Thomas Jefferson's Flower Garden at Monticello,* 3rd ed. (Charlottesville, VA: University of Virginia Press, 1971).

68 S. Crumpe, *An Inquiry into the Nature and Properties of Opium: Wherein Its Component Principles, Mode of Operation, and Use or Abuse in Particular Diseases, Are Experimentally Investigated, and the Opinions of Former Authors on These Points Impartially Examined* (London: G. G. and J. Robinson, 1793).

69 Ibid.

70 F. W. Sertürner, "Über das Morphium, eine neue salzfähige Grundlage, und die Mekonsäure, als Hauptbestandteile des Opiums," *Annalen der Physik* 25 (1817), 56–90; Macht, "History of Opium."

71 Jaime Wisniak, "Pierre-Jean Robiquet," *Educación Química* 24 (S1: March 2013), 139–49; P.-J. Robiquet, "Nouvelles observations sur les principaux produits de l'opium," *Ann. Chim. Phys.* 51:2 (1832), 225–67.

72 C. R. A. Wright, "On the Action of Organic Acids and their Anhydrides on the Natural Alkaloids," *Journal of the Chemical Society* 27 (1874), 1031–43.

73 Chemical Heritage Foundation, "Felix Hoffmann," www.chemheritage.org/historical -profile/felix-hoffmann. Accessed September 10, 2017.

74 R. Askwith, "How Aspirin Turned Hero," *Sunday Times* (London), September 13, 1998.

75 M. Manges, "A Second Report on Therapeutics of Heroin," *New York Medical Journal* 71, 51; Heinrich Dreser, "Heroin: A New Derivative of Morphine," *Le Bul. Méd.* 80 (October

5, 1898); G. Strube, "Mittheilung über therapeutische Versuche mit Heroin," *Klinische Wochenschrift* 1898, 38.

76 Manges, "Second Report."

77 Thomas Brown, "The Hypodermic or Subcutaneous Syringe," in *Alexander Wood: A sketch of His Life and Work* (Edinburgh: Macniven & Wallace, 1886), 107–114.

78 Yangwen Zheng, "The Art of Alchemists, Sex, and Court Ladies," in *The Social Life of Opium in China* (Cambridge, UK: Cambridge University Press, 2005).

79 F. Dikötter, L. Laaman, and Z. Xun, *Narcotic Culture: A History of Drugs in China* (Chicago: University of Chicago Press, 2004), 34.

80 Anthony S. Wohl, *Endangered Lives: Public Health in Victorian Britain* (Cambridge, MA: Harvard University Press, 1983).

81 Jonathan Minton, Jane Parkinson, James Lewsey, Janet Bouttell, and Gerry McCartney, "Drug Related Deaths in Scotland," Open Science Framework, July 25, 2017, doi:10.17605/OSF.IO/ECBPN.

82 Dan Baum, "Legalize It All: How to Win the War on Drugs," *Harper's Magazine*, April 2016.

83 American Civil Liberties Union, "Finding 4: Blacks and Whites Use Marijuana at Similar Rates," *The War on Marijuana in Black and White,* June 2013, 21.

84 Julie Netherland and Helena Hansen, White opioids: Pharmaceutical race and the war on drugs that wasn't," *BioSocieties* 12:2 (June 2017), 217–38.

85 Macht, "History of Opium."

86 European Monitoring Centre for Drugs and Drug Addiction, "Fentanyl Drug Profile," www.emcdda.europa.eu/publications/drug-profiles/fentanyl#pharmacology; D. Algren, C. Monteilh, C. Rubin, et al., "Fentanyl-Associated Fatalities among Illicit Drug Users in Wayne County, Michigan (July 2005–May 2006)," *Journal of Medical Toxicology* 9:1 (March 2013), 106–15.

87 DrugBank Database, "Carfentanil," www.drugbank.ca/drugs/DB01535.

88 National Institute on Drug Abuse, "Fentanyl," www.drugabuse.gov/publications/drugfacts/fentanyl.

89 PubChem Compound Database, "Carfentanil," http://pubchem.ncbi.nlm.nih.gov/compound/62156. Accessed September 13, 2017.

90 C. B. Pert and S. H. Snyder, "Opiate Receptor: Demonstration in Nervous Tissue," *Science* 179:4077 (March 1973), 1011–14.

91 J. Hughes, T. W. Smith, H. W. Kosterlitz, L. A. Fothergill, B. A. Morgan, and H. R. Morris, "Identification of Two Related Pentapeptides from the Brain with Potent Opiate Agonist Activity," *Nature* 258:5536 (December 1975), 577–80; R. Simantov and S. H. Snyder, "Morphine-like Peptides in Mammalian Brain: Isolation, Structure Elucidation, and Interactions with the Opiate Receptor," *Proceedings of the National Academy of Sciences of the United States of America* 73:7 (July 1976), 2515–19.

92   H. Boecker, T. Sprenger, M. E. Spilker, G. Henriksen, M. Koppenhoefer, K. J. Wagner, M. Valet, A. Berthele, and T. R. Tolle, "The Runner's High: Opioidergic Mechanisms in the Human Brain," *Cerebral Cortex* 18:11 (November 2008), 2523–31.

93   M. Palkovits, "The Brain and the Pain: Neurotransmitters and Neuronal Pathways of Pain Perception and Response," *Orv. Hetil.* 141:41 (October 8, 2000), 2231–39.

94   J. C. Meunier, C. Mollereau, L. Toll, C. Suaudeau, C. Moisand, P. Alvinerie, J. L. Butour, J. C. Guillemot, P. Ferrara, and B. Monsarrat, "Isolation and Structure of the Endogenous Agonist of Opioid Receptor-Like ORL1 Receptor," *Nature* 377:6549 (October 1995), 532–35.

95   C. W. Stevens, K. K. Martin, and B. W. Stahlheber, "Nociceptin Produces Antinociception after Spinal Administration in Amphibians," *Pharmacology, Biochemistry, and Behavior* 91:3 (2009), 436–40.

96   A. Hernández, M. A. Sola, B. Domínguez, M. I. Rochera, P. Bascuñana, and V. Gancedo, "Is Morphine Still the Analgesic of Choice in Acute Myocardial Infarction?" *Rev. Esp. Anestesiol. Reanim.* 55:1 (January 2008), 32–39; P. E. Molina, "Opioids and Opiates: Analgesia with Cardiovascular, Haemodynamic and Immune Implications in Critical Illness," *Journal of Internal Medicine* 259 (2006), 138–54.

97   J. K. Zubieta, Y. R. Smith, J. A. Bueller, Y. Xu, M. R. Kilbourn, D. M. Jewett, C. R. Meyer, R. A. Koeppe, and C. S. Stohler, "Regional Mu Opioid Receptor Regulation of Sensory and Affective Dimensions of Pain," *Science* 293 (2001), 311–15.

98   R. Abs, J. Verhelst, J. Maeyaert, J. P. Van Buyten, F. Opsomer, H. Adriaensen, Jan Verlooy, Tony Van Havenbergh, Mike Smet, and Kristien Van Acker, "Endocrine Consequences of Long-Term Intrathecal Administration of Opioids," *J. Clin. Endocrinol. Metab.* 85 (2000), 2215–22.

99   J. Tiihonen, M. Lehti, M. Aaltonen, et al., "Psychotropic Drugs and Homicide: A Prospective Cohort Study from Finland," *World Psychiatry* 14:2 (2015), 245–47.

100 Robert G. Morris, Michael TenEyck, J. C. Barnes, and Tomislav V. Kovandzic, "The Effect of Medical Marijuana Laws on Crime: Evidence from State Panel Data, 1990–2006," *PLoS ONE* 9:3, e92816.

101 Charles T. Tart, "Marijuana Intoxication: Common Experiences," *Nature* 226:5247 (May 1970), 701–4.

102 J. Volpi-Abadie, A. M. Kaye, and A. D. Kaye, "Serotonin Syndrome," *The Ochsner Journal* 13:4 (2013), 533–40.

103 Ibid.

104 A. S. Lee and S. M. Twigg, "Opioid-Induced Secondary Adrenal Insufficiency Presenting as Hypercalcaemia," *Endocrinology, Diabetes & Metabolism Case Reports* 2015:150035; C. Lee, S. Ludwig, and D. R. Duerksen, "Low-Serum Cortisol Associated with Opioid Use: Case Report and Review of the Literature," *Endocrinologist* 12 (2002), 5–8.

105 J. H. Mendelson, J. Ellingboe, J. C. Kuehnle, and N. K. Mello, "Heroin and Naltrexone Effects on Pituitary-Gonadal Hormones in Man: Interaction of Steroid Feedback Effects, Tolerance and Supersensitivity," *J. Pharmacol. Exp. Ther.* 214 (1980), 503–6.

106 H. W. Daniell, "Opioid Endocrinopathy in Women Consuming Prescribed Sustained-Action Opioids for Control of Nonmalignant Pain," *J. Pain* 9 (2008), 28–36.

107 P. W. Kalivas and N. D. Volkow, "The Neural Basis of Addiction: A Pathology of Motivation and Choice," *American Journal of Psychiatry* 162:8 (August, 2005), 1403–13.

108 Secretary-General of the United Nations. Single Convention on Narcotic Drugs (of 1961). No. 14152. Signed March 30, 1961. In force August 8, 1975. Parties: 185.

109 Daniel M. Perrine, *The Chemistry of Mind-Altering Drugs* (Washington, DC: American Chemical Society, 1997).

110 James C. Anthony, Lynn A. Warner, and Ronald C. Kessler, "Comparative Epidemiology of Dependence on Tobacco, Alcohol, Controlled Substances, and Inhalants: Basic Findings from the National Comorbidity Survey," *Experimental and Clinical Psychopharmacology* 2:3 (1994), 244–68.

111 American Psychiatric Association, *Diagnostic and Statistical Manual of Mental Disorders,* 5th ed. (*DSM-5*): "Opioid-Related Disorders: 540" (Arlington, VA: American Psychiatric Publishing, 2013).

112 Ibid. Opioid withdrawal: 547.

113 Jean Cocteau, *Opium* (London: Peter Owens Publishers, 1930), 14.

114 Seal et al., "Predictors and Prevention of Nonfatal Overdose."

115 U.S. CDC, "Provisional Counts of Overdose Deaths."

116 M. S. Lee, "Molecular Clock Calibrations and Metazoan Divergence Dates," *J. Mol. Evol.* 49 (1999), 385–91; John M. McPartland and Patty Pruitt, "Sourcing the Code: Searching for the Evolutionary Origins of Cannabinoid Receptors, Vanilloid Receptors, and Anandamide," *Journal of Cannabis Therapeutics* 2:1 (2002); Susanne Dreborg, Görel Sundström, Tomas A. Larsson, and Dan Larhammar, "Evolution of Vertebrate Opioid Receptors," *PNAS* 105:40, 15487–92.

117 Y. Gaoni and R. Mechoulam, "Isolation, Structure and Partial Synthesis of an Active Constituent of Hashish," *J. Am. Chem. Soc.* 86:620 (1964), 1646–47.

118 W. A. Devane, F. A. Dysarz III, M. R. Johnson, L. S. Melvin, and A. C. Howlett, "Determination and Characterization of a Cannabinoid Receptor in Rat Brain," *Mol. Pharmacol.* 34:5 (November 1988), 605–13.

119 S. Munro, K. L. Thomas, and M. Abu-Shaar, "Molecular Characterization of a Peripheral Receptor for Cannabinoids," *Nature* 365 (1993), 61–65.

120 W. A. Devane, L. Hanus, A. Breuer, R. G. Pertwee, L. A. Stevenson, G. Griffin, D. Gibson, A. Mandelbaum, A. Etinger, and R. Mechoulam, "Isolation and Structure of a Brain Constituent that Binds to the Cannabinoid Receptor," *Science* 258 (1992), 1946–49.

121 E. B. Russo and G. W. Guy, "A Tale of Two Cannabinoids: The Therapeutic Rationale for Combining Tetrahydrocannabinol and Cannabidiol," *Med. Hypotheses* 66 (2006), 234–46; E. B. Russo, "Taming THC: Potential Cannabis Synergy and Phytocannabinoid-Terpenoid Entourage Effects," *British Journal of Pharmacology* 163:7 (2011), 1344–64; Christian D.

Schubart et al., "Cannabis with High Cannabidiol Content Is Associated with Fewer Psychotic Experiences," *Schizophrenia Research* 130:1, 216–21; R. Gallily, Z. Yekhtin, and L. O. Hanuš, "Overcoming the Bell-Shaped Dose-Response of Cannabidiol by Using Cannabis Extract Enriched in Cannabidiol," *Pharmacology & Pharmacy* 6 (2015), 75–85.

122 N. Agarwal, P. Pacher, I. Tegeder, et al., "Cannabinoids Mediate Analgesia Largely Via Peripheral Type 1 Cannabinoid Receptors in Nociceptors, *Nature Neuroscience* 10:7 (2007), 870–79; J. M. Walker and A. G. Hohmann, "Cannabinoid Mechanisms of Pain Suppression," *Handb. Exp. Pharmacol.* 168 (2005), 509–54.

123 Agarwal et al., "Cannabinoids Mediate Analgesia."

124 C. C. Felder, K. E. Joyce, E. M. Briley, J. Mansouri, K. Mackie, O. Blond, Y. Lai, A. L. Ma, and R.L. Mitchell, "Comparison of the Pharmacology and Signal Transduction of the Human Cannabinoid CB1 and CB2 Receptors," *Mol. Pharmacol.* 48:3 (September 1995), 443–50.

125 J. M. McPartland, M. Glass, and R. G. Pertwee, "Meta-analysis of Cannabinoid Ligand Binding Affinity and Receptor Distribution: Interspecies Differences," *British Journal of Pharmacology* 152:5 (2007), 583–93.

126 Katie Kingwell, "Analgesics: Pain Control at the Periphery," *Nature Reviews Drug Discovery* 9 (November 2010), 839; J. R. Clapper, G. Moreno-Sanz, R. Russo, et al., "Anandamide Suppresses Pain Initiation through a Peripheral Endocannabinoid Mechanism," *Nature Neuroscience* 13:10 (2010), 1265–70.

127 K. Starowicz, W. Makuch, M. Osikowicz, F. Piscitelli, S. Petrosino, V. Di Marzo, and B. Przewlocka, "Spinal Anandamide Produces Analgesia in Neuropathic Rats: Possible CB(1)- and TRPV1-Mediated Mechanisms," *Neuropharmacology* 62:4 (March 2012), 1746–55.

128 L. Chen, J. Zhang, F. Li, Y. Qiu, L. Wang, Y. H. Li, J. Shi, H. L. Pan, and M. Li, "Endogenous Anandamide and Cannabinoid Receptor-2 Contribute to Electroacupuncture Analgesia in Rats," *J. Pain* 10:7 (July 2009), 732–39; S. E. O'Sullivan and D. A. Kendall, "Cannabinoid Activation of Peroxisome Proliferator-Activated Receptors: Potential for Modulation of Inflammatory Disease," *Immunobiology* 215:8 (August 2010), 611–16.

129 Karen A. Willoughby, Sandra F. Moore, Billy R. Martin, and Earl F. Ellis, "The Biodisposition and Metabolism of Anandamide in Mice," *Journal of Pharmacology and Experimental Therapeutics* 282:1 (July 1997), 243–47.

130 Benjamin F. Cravatt, Kristin Demarest, Matthew P. Patricelli, Michael H. Bracey, Dan K. Giang, Billy R. Martin, and Aron H. Lichtman, "Supersensitivity to Anandamide and Enhanced Endogenous Cannabinoid Signaling in Mice Lacking Fatty Acid Amide Hydrolase, *PNAS* 98:16, 9371–76.

131 L. B. Resstel, R. F. Tavares, S. F. Lisboa, S. R. Joca, F. M. Corrêa, and F. S. Guimarães, "5-HT$_{1A}$ Receptors Are Involved in the Cannabidiol-Induced Attenuation of Behavioural and Cardiovascular Responses to Acute Restraint Stress in Rats," *Br. J. Pharmacol.* 156:1 (January 2009), 181–88; D. Parolaro, N. Realini, D. Vigano, C. Guidali, and T. Rubino,

"The Endocannabinoid System and Psychiatric Disorders," *Exp. Neurol.* 224:1 (July 2010), 3–14; J. A. Crippa, A. W. Zuardi, and J. E. Hallak, "Therapeutical Use of the Cannabinoids in Psychiatry," *Rev. Bras. Psiquiatr.* 32 (May 2010), suppl. 1, S56–66.

132 Resstel et al., "5-HT$_{1A}$ Receptors."

133 E. Nalivaiko, Y. Ootsuka, and W. W. Blessing, "Activation of 5-HT$_{1A}$ Receptors in the Medullary Raphe Reduces Cardiovascular Changes Elicited by Acute Psychological and Inflammatory Stresses in Rabbits," *Am. J. Physiol. Regul. Integr. Comp. Physiol.* 289:2 (2005), R596–R604.

134 G. A. Kennett, C. T. Dourish, and G. Curzon, "Antidepressant-like Action of 5-HT$_{1A}$ Agonists and Conventional Antidepressants in an Animal Model of Depression," *European Journal of Pharmacology* 134:3 (February 24, 1987), 265–74.

135 N. K. Popova et al., "Involvement of the 5-HT$_{1A}$ and 5-HT$_{1B}$ Serotonergic Receptor Subtypes in Sexual Arousal in Male Mice," *Psychoneuroendocrinology* 27:5 (July 2002), 609–18.

136 Sarah Rosenthaler, Birgit Pöhn, Caroline Kolmanz, Chi Nguyen Huu, Christopher Krewenka, Alexandra Huber, Barbara Kranner, Wolf-Dieter Rausch, and Rudolf Moldzio, "Differences in Receptor Binding Affinity of Several Phytocannabinoids Do Not Explain Their Effects on Neural Cell Cultures," *Neurotoxicology and Teratology* 46 (2014), 49–56.

137 Cravatt et al., "Supersensitivity to Anandamide."

138 M. Kathmann, K. Flau, A. Redmer, C. Tränkle, and E. Schlicker, "Cannabidiol Is an Allosteric Modulator at Mu- and Delta-Opioid Receptors," *Naunyn Schmiedebergs Arch. Pharmacol.* 372:5 (February 2006), 354–61.

139 T. Iuvone, G. Esposito, D. De Filippis, C. Scuderi, and L. Steardo, "Cannabidiol: A Promising Drug for Neurodegenerative Disorders?" *CNS Neurosci. Ther.* 15:1 (Winter 2009), 65–75; Carol Hamelink, Aidan Hampson, David A. Wink, Lee E. Eiden, and Robert L. Eskay, "Comparison of Cannabidiol, Antioxidants, and Diuretics in Reversing Binge Ethanol-Induced Neurotoxicity," *JPET* 314:2 (August 2005), 780–88.

140 L. De Petrocellis, A. Ligresti, A. S. Moriello, et al., "Effects of Cannabinoids and Cannabinoid-Enriched Cannabis Extracts on TRP Channels and Endocannabinoid Metabolic Enzymes," *British Journal of Pharmacology* 163:7 (2011), 1479–94.

141 T. Bisogno, L. Hanus, L. De Petrocellis, S. Tchilibon, D. E. Ponde, I. Brandi, et al., "Molecular Targets for Cannabidiol and Its Synthetic Analogues: Effect on Vanilloid VR1 Receptors and on the Cellular Uptake and Enzymatic Hydrolysis of Anandamide," *Br. J. Pharmacol.* 134 (2001), 845–52.

142 B. Costa, G. Giagnoni, C. Franke, A. E. Trovato, and M. Colleoni, "Vanilloid TRPV1 Receptor Mediates the Antihyperalgesic Effect of the Nonpsychoactive Cannabinoid, Cannabidiol, in a Rat Model of Acute Inflammation," *British Journal of Pharmacology* 143:2 (2004), 247–50; R. Ramachandran, E. Hyun, L. Zhao, T. K. Lapointe, K. Chapman, C. L. Hirota, S. Ghosh, et al., "TRPM8 Activation Attenuates Inflammatory Responses in Mouse Models of Colitis," *Proc. Natl. Acad. Sci. USA* 110 (2013), 7476–81.

143 T. Maeda and S. Kishioka, "PPAR and Pain," *Int. Rev. Neurobiol.* 85 (2009), 165–77.

144 McPartland et al., "Meta-analysis of Cannabinoid Ligand Binding Affinity."

145 R. G. Pertwee, "Cannabinoid receptors and pain," *Prog. Neurobiol.* 63 (2001), 569–611; N. Agarwal, P. Pacher, I. Tegeder, F. Amaya, C. E. Constantin, G. J. Brenner, T. Rubino, et al., "Cannabinoids Mediate Analgesia Largely Via Peripheral Type 1 Cannabinoid Receptors in Nociceptors," *Nat. Neurosci.* 10 (2007), 870–79; W. P. Farquhar-Smith, M. Egertová, E. J. Bradbury, S. B. McMahon, A. S. Rice, and M. R. Elphick, "Cannabinoid CB(1) Receptor Expression in Rat Spinal Cord," *Mol. Cell. Neurosci* 15 (2000), 510–21.

146 M. D. Jhaveri, D. R. Sagar, S. J. Elmes, D. A. Kendall, and V. Chapman, "Cannabinoid CB2 Receptor-Mediated Anti-nociception in Models of Acute and Chronic Pain," *Mol. Neurobiol.* 36 (2007), 26–35; J. C. Ashton and M. Glass, "The Cannabinoid CB2 Receptor as a Target for Inflammation-Dependent Neurodegeneration," *Current Neuropharmacology* 5:2 (2007), 73–80; D. Ziring, B. Wei, P. Velazquez, M. Schrage, N. E. Buckley, and J. Braun, "Formation of B and T Cell Subsets Require the Cannabinoid Receptor CB2," *Immunogenetics.* 58 (2006), 714–25.

147 W. Notcutt, M. Price, A. Miller, et al., "Initial Experiences with Medicinal Extracts of Cannabis for Chronic Pain: Results from 34 ▨N of 1▨ Studies," *Anaesthesia* 59 (2004), 440–52; M. A. Ware, T. Wang, S. Shapiro, and J. P. Collet, "Cannabis for the Management of Pain: Assessment of Safety Study (COMPASS)," *Journal of Pain* 16:12 (2015), 1233–42.

148 D. McHugh, "GPR18 in Microglia: Implications for the CNS and Endocannabinoid System Signalling," *British Journal of Pharmacology* 167:8 (2012), 1575–82.

149 Maeda and Kishioka, "PPAR and Pain"; M. Brusberg, S. Arvidsson, D. Kang, H. Larsson, E. Lindström, and V. Martinez, "CB1 Receptors Mediate the Analgesic Effects of Cannabinoids on Colorectal Distension-Induced Visceral Pain in Rodents," *J. Neurosci.* 29:5 (February 4, 2009), 1554–64.

150 Kathmann et al., "Cannabidiol Is an Allosteric Modulator."

151 Y. Tamura, Y. Iwasaki, M. Narukawa, and T. Watanabe, "Ingestion of Cinnamaldehyde, a TRPA1 Agonist, Reduces Visceral Fats in Mice Fed a High-Fat and High-Sucrose Diet," *J. Nutr. Sci. Vitaminol.* (Tokyo) 58:1 (2012), 9–13; A. N. Akopian, N. B. Ruparel, N. A. Jeske, A. Patwardhan, and K. M. Hargreaves, "Role of Ionotropic Cannabinoid Receptors in Peripheral Antinociception and Antihyperalgesia," *Trends Pharmacol. Sci.* 30 (2009), 79–84; W. J. Winchester, K. Gore, S. Glatt, W. Petit, J. C. Gardiner, K. Conlon, M. Postlethwaite, et al., "Inhibition of TRPM8 Channels Reduces Pain in the Cold Pressor Test in Humans," *Pharmacol. Exp. Ther.* 351:2 (November 2014), 259–69.

152 E. Small and H. D. Beckstead, "Cannabinoid Phenotypes in *Cannabis sativa*," *Nature* 245 (1973), 147–48; E. Small and H. D. Beckstead, "Common Cannabinoid Phenotypes in 350 Stocks of Cannabis," *Lloydia* 36 (1973), 144–65.

153 Karl W. Hillig and Paul G. Mahlberg, "A Chemotaxonomic Analysis of Cannabinoid Variation in Cannabis (Cannabaceae)," *Am. J. Bot.* 91:6 (June 2004), 966–75.

154 G. Fournier, C. Richez-Dumanois, J. Duvezin, J.-P. Mathieu, and M. Paris, "Identification of a New Chemotype in *Cannabis sativa:* Cannabigerol-Dominant Plants, Biogenetic and Agronomic Prospects," *Plant. Med.* 53 (1987), 277–80.

155 G. Mandolino and A. Carboni, "Potential of Marker Assisted Selection in Hemp Genetic Improvement," *Euphytica* 140 (2004), 107–20.

156 Z. D. Cooper, S. D. Comer, and M. Haney, "Comparison of the Analgesic Effects of Dronabinol and Smoked Marijuana in Daily Marijuana Smokers," *Neuropsychopharmacology* 38:10 (2013), 1984–92.

157 S. Narang, D. Gibson, A. D. Wasan, E. L. Ross, E. Michna, S. S. Nedeljkovic, and R. N. Jamison, "Efficacy of Dronabinol as an Adjuvant Treatment for Chronic Pain Patients on Opioid Therapy," *J. Pain* 9:3 (March 2008), 254–64.

158 A. Bisaga, M. A. Sullivan, A. Glass, et al., "The Effects of Dronabinol During Detoxification and the Initiation of Treatment With Extended Release Naltrexone," *Drug and Alcohol Dependence* 154 (2015), 38–45.

159 "The Strongest Strains on Earth," *High Times,* May 2017. High-performance liquid chromatography lab testing done by Canna Safe Analytics, Murrieta, CA.

160 Ibid.

161 Ibid.

162 Russo et al., "A Tale of Two Cannabinoids"; Russo, "Taming THC"; Schubart et al., "Cannabis with High Cannabidiol Content;" Gallily et al., "Overcoming the Bell-Shaped Dose-Response."

163 Russell K. Portenoy, Elena Doina Ganae-Motan, Silvia Allende, Ronald Yanagihara, Lauren Shaiova, Sharon Weinstein, Robert McQuade, et al., "Nabiximols for Opioid-Treated Cancer Patients With Poorly-Controlled Chronic Pain: A Randomized, Placebo-Controlled, Graded-Dose Trial," *Journal of Pain* 13:5 (May 2012), 438–49.

164 M. E. Lynch and F. Campbell, "Cannabinoids for Treatment of Chronic Noncancer Pain: A Systematic Review of Randomized Trials," *British Journal of Clinical Pharmacology* 72:5 (2011), 735–44.

165 Bayer and GW Pharmaceutical, "Sativex Oromucosal Spray." Patient information leaflet. May 20, 2015.

166 "The Strongest Strains on Earth," 80.

167 Ibid.

168 Antony Paul Hornby, Hayley's Comet, patent CA2737447A1, filed April 27, 2011.

169 Lion Fire (flower), batch number PA11686-688, tested by Pure Analytics, Santa Rosa, CA, October 10, 2016.

170 .GW Pharmaceuticals, "Epidiolex," www.gwpharm.com/epilepsy-patients-caregivers/patients.

171 Ibid.

172 Mateus Machado Bergamaschi, Regina Helena Costa Queiroz, José Alexandre S. Crippa, and Antonio Waldo Zuardi, "Safety and Side Effects of Cannabidiol, a Cannabis sativa Constituent," *Current Drug Safety* 6:4 (2011).

173 G. Jones and R. G. Pertwee, "A Metabolic Interaction In Vivo between Cannabidiol and 1-Tetrahydrocannabinol," *Br. J. Pharmacol.* 45:2 (1972), 375–77.

174 M. D. Srivastava, B. I. Srivastava, and B. Brouhard, "D9-Tetrahydrocannabinol and Cannabidiol Alter Cytokine Production by Human Immune Cells, *Immunopharmacology* 40:3 (1998), 179–85.

175 ProCon.org, "Deaths from Marijuana v. 17 FDA-Approved Drugs: Jan. 1, 1997 to June 30, 2005," July 8, 2009, http://goo.gl/ygFFby; U.S. Department of Health and Human Services, Substance Abuse and Mental Health Services Administration, *Mortality Data from the Drug Abuse Warning Network, 2002* (Rockville, MD: NCADI, 2002). See p. 18, table H, and p. 24 where it states "marijuana is rarely the only drug involved in a drug abuse death. Thus, in many MSA's, the proportion of marijuana involved cases labeled as 'one drug' (i.e., marijuana only) will be zero or nearly zero."

176 CDC, "Smoking-Attributable Mortality, Years of Potential Life Lost, and Productivity Losses—United States, 2000–2004," *MMWR* 57:45 (November 14, 2008), 1226–28.

177 CDC, "Alcohol-Attributable Deaths and Years of Potential Life Lost—United States, 2001," *MMWR* 53:37 (September 24, 2004), 866–70.

178 ProCon.org, "Deaths from Marijuana."

179 A. De Laurentiis, J. Fernández-Solari, C. Mohn, M. Zorrilla Zubilete, and V. Rettori, "Endocannabinoid System Participates in Neuroendocrine Control of Homeostasis," *Neuroimmunomodulation* 17:3 (2010), 153–56.

180 J. Yang, Y. Yang, J. M. Chen, W. Y. Liu, C. H. Wang, and B. C. Lin, "Central Oxytocin Enhances Antinociception in the Rat," *Peptides* 28:5 (May 2007), 1113–19.

181 A. Vitalo, J. Fricchione, M. Casali, Y. Berdichevsky, E. A. Hoge, S. L. Rauch, F. Berthiaume, et al., "Nest-Making and Oxytocin Comparably Promote Wound Healing in Isolation-Reared Rats." *PLoS One* 4:5 (2009), e5523.

182 M. Kosfeld, M. Heinrichs, P. J. Zak, U. Fischbacher, and E. Fehr, "Oxytocin Increases Trust in Humans," *Nature* 435:7042 (June 2, 2005), 673–76.

183 P. J. Zak, A. A. Stanton, and S. Ahmadi, "Oxytocin Increases Generosity in Humans," *PLoS One* 2:11 (November 7, 2007), e1128.

184 M. H. Meier, A. Caspi, A. Ambler, H. Harrington, R. Houts, R. S. Keefe, K. McDonald, et al., "Persistent Cannabis Users Show Neuropsychological Decline from Childhood to Midlife," *Proc. Natl. Acad. Sci. USA* 109:40 (October 2, 2012), E2657–64.

185 P. Silva and W. Stanton, *From Child to Adult: The Dunedin Multidisciplinary Health and Development Study* (Oxford, UK: Oxford University Press, 1996).

186 M. Hashibe, H. Morgenstern, Y. Cui, D. P. Tashkin, Z. F. Zhang, W. Cozen, T. M. Mack, and S. Greenland, "Marijuana Use and the Risk of Lung and Upper Aerodigestive Tract Cancers: Results of a Population-Based Case-Control Study," *Cancer Epidemiol. Biomarkers Prev.* 15:10 (October 2006), 1829–34.

187 Karl-Christian Bergmann, "Dronabinol—eine mögliche neue erapie- option bei COPD-Patienten mit pulmonaler Kachexie," paper presented at the 2005 Conference of the German Society for Pneumology, Berlin, March 17, 2005.

188 S. J. Williams, J. P. Hartley, and J. D. Graham, "Bronchodilator Effect of Delta1-Tetra-hydrocannabinol Administered by Aerosol of Asthmatic Patients," *Thorax* 31:6 (1976), 720–23; D. P. Tashkin, S. Reiss, B. J. Shapiro, B. Calvarese, J. L. Olsen, and J. W. Lodge, "Bronchial Effects of Aerosolized Delta 9-Tetrahydrocannabinol in Healthy and Asthmatic Subjects," *Am. Rev. Respir. Dis.* 115:1 (January 1977), 57–65; J. P. Hartley, S. G. Nogrady, and A. Seaton, "Bronchodilator Effect Of Delta1-Tetrahydrocannabinol," *Br. J. Clin. Pharmacol.* 5:6 (June 1978), 523–25.

189 K. Hayakawa, K. Mishima, K. Abe, N. Hasebe, F. Takamatsu, H. Yasuda, T. Ikeda, et al., "Cannabidiol Prevents Infarction via the Non-CB1 Cannabinoid Receptor Mechanism," *Neuroreport* 15:15 (October 25, 2004), 2381–85; Y. A. Shmist, I. Goncharov, M. Eichler, V. Shneyvays, A. Isaac, Z. Vogel, and A. Shainberg, "Delta-9-Tetrahydrocannabinol Protects Cardiac Cells from Hypoxia via CB2 Receptor Activation and Nitric Oxide Production," *Mol. Cell Biochem.* 283:1–2 (February 2006), 75–83; D. Lamontagne, P. Lépicier, C. Lagneux, and J. F. Bouchard, "The Endogenous Cardiac Cannabinoid System: A New Protective Mechanism against Myocardial Ischemia," *Arch. Mal Coeur Vaiss.* 99:3 (March 2006), 242–46; Ronen Durst, Haim Danenberg, Ruth Gallily, Raphael Mechoulam, Keren Meir, Etty Grad, Ronen Beeri, et al., "Cannabidiol, a Nonpsychoactive Cannabis Constituent, Protects against Myocardial Ischemic Reperfusion Injury," *Am. J. Physiol. Heart Circ. Physiol.* 293 (2007), H3602–7; J. C. Ashton and P. F. Smith, "Cannabinoids and Cardiovascular Disease: The Outlook for Clinical Treatments," *Curr. Vasc. Pharmacol.* 5:3 (July 2007), 175–85; Resstel et al., "5-HT receptors are involved"; S. K. Walsh, C. Y. Hepburn, K. A. Kane, and C. L. Wainwright, "Acute Administration of Cannabidiol In Vivo Suppresses Ischaemia-Induced Cardiac Arrhythmias and Reduces Infarct Size When Given at Reperfusion," *British Journal of Pharmacology* 160:5 (2010), 1234–42; M. Waldman, E. Hochhauser, M. Fishbein, D. Aravot, A. Shainberg, and Y. Sarne, "An Ultralow Dose of Tetrahydrocannabinol Provides Cardioprotection," *Biochem. Pharmacol.* 85:11 (June 1, 2013), 1626–33; Y. Lu, B. C. Akinwumi, Z. Shao, and H. D. Anderson, "Ligand Activation of Cannabinoid Receptors Attenuates Hypertrophy of Neonatal Rat Cardiomyocytes," *J. Cardiovasc. Pharmacol.* 64:5 (November 2014), 420–30; N. Vin-Raviv, T. Akinyemiju, Q. Meng, S. Sakhuja, and R. Hayward, "Marijuana Use and Inpatient Outcomes among Hospitalized Patients: Analysis of the Nationwide Inpatient Sample Database," *Cancer Med.* 6:1 (January 2017), 320–29; R. Kaur, S. R. Ambwani, and S. Singh, "Endocannabinoid System: A Multi-Facet Therapeutic Target," *Curr. Clin. Pharmacol.* 11:2 (2016), 110–17.

190 R. Secades-Villa, O. Garcia-Rodríguez, C. J. Jin, S. Wang, and C. Blanco, "Probability and Predictors of the Cannabis Gateway Effect: A National Study," *International Journal of Drug Policy* 26:2 (2015), 135–42.

191 Thomas J. O'Connell and Ché B. Bou-Matar, "Long-Term Marijuana Users Seeking Medical Cannabis in California (2001–2007): Demographics, Social Characteristics, Patterns of Cannabis and Other Drug Use of 4,117 Applicants," *Harm Reduction Journal* 4:16 (2007).

192 G. R. Thompson, H. Rosenkrantz, U. H. Schaeppi, and M. C. Braude, "Comparison of Acute Oral Toxicity of Cannabinoids in Rats, Dogs and Monkeys," *Toxicol. Appl. Pharmacol.* 25 (1973), 363–72.

193 Gregory T. Carter, Patrick Weydt, Muraco Kyashna-Tocha, and Donald Abrams, "Medicinal Cannabis: Rational Guidelines for Dosing," *IDrugs* 7:5 (May 2004), 464–70; A. F. Manini, G. Yiannoulos, M. M. Bergamaschi, et al., "Safety and Pharmacokinetics of Oral Cannabidiol When Administered Concomitantly with Intravenous Fentanyl in Humans," *Journal of Addiction Medicine* 9:3 (2015), 204–10.

194 S. Walther, R. Mahlberg, U. Eichmann, and D. Kunz, "Delta-9-Tetrahydrocannabinol for Nighttime Agitation in Severe Dementia," *Psychopharmacology* (Berl). 185:4 (May 2006), 524–28.

195 Mean Ki at human CB1 is 239.2nM, Mean Ki 25nM at CB1: McPartland et al., "Meta-analysis of Cannabinoid Ligand Binding Affinity."

196 P. F. Sumariwalla, R. Gallily, S. Tchilibon, E. Fride, R. Mechoulam, and M. Feldmann, "A Novel Synthetic, Nonpsychoactive Cannabinoid Acid (HU-320) with Antiinflammatory Properties in Murine Collagen-Induced Arthritis," *Arthritis Rheum.* 50:3 (2004), 985–998; B. Costa, A. E. Trovato, F. Comelli, G. Giagnoni, and M. Colleoni, "The Nonpsychoactive Cannabis Constituent Cannabidiol Is an Orally Effective Therapeutic Agent in Rat Chronic Inflammatory and Neuropathic Pain," *Eur. J. Pharmacol.* 556:1–3 (2007), 75–83.

197 H. K. Beecher, "Relationship of Significance of Wound to Pain Experienced," *JAMA* 161:17 (August 1956), 1609–13.

198 G. L. Moseley, T. J. Parsons, and C. Spence, "Visual Distortion of a Limb Modulates the Pain and Swelling Evoked by Movement," *Curr. Biol.* 18:22 (November 2008), R1047–48.

199 H. S. Smith and P. D. Meek, "Pain Responsiveness to Opioids: Central Versus Peripheral Neuropathic Pain," *J. Opioid Manag.* 7:5 (September–October 2011), 391–400; S. Arnér and B. A. Meyerson, "Lack of Analgesic Effect Of opioids on Neuropathic and Idiopathic Forms of Pain," *Pain* 33:1 (April 1988), 11–23.

200 Harold Merskey and Nikolai Bogduk, *Classification of Chronic Pain: Description of Chronic Pain Syndromes and Definition of Pain Terms* (Seattle: IASP Press, 1994); I. D. Meng, B. H. Manning, W. J. Martin, and H. L. Fields, "An Analgesia Circuit Activated by Cannabinoids," *Nature* 395:6700 (September 24, 1998), 381–83; Jack Rocky-Jay Rivers and John Clive Ashton, "The Development of Cannabinoid CBII Receptor Agonists for the Treatment of Central Neuropathies," *Central Nervous System Agents in Medicinal Chemistry* 10 (2010), 47–64; D. J. Rog, T. Nurmiko, T. Friede, et al., "Randomized Controlled Trial of

Cannabis-Based Medicine in Central Neuropathic Pain Due to Multiple Sclerosis," *Neurology* 65 (2005), 812–19; D. T. Wade, P. Robson, H. House, et al., "A Preliminary Controlled Study to Determine Whether Whole-Plant Cannabis Extracts Can Improve Intractable Neurogenic Symptoms," *Clin. Rehabil.* 17:1 (2003), 18–26; J. S. Berman, C. Symonds, and R. Birch, "Efficacy of Two Cannabis-Based Medicinal Extracts for Relief of Central Neuropathic Pain from Brachial Plexus Avulsion: Results of a Randomised Controlled Trial," *Pain* 112:3 (2004), 299–306.

201 Smith et al., "Pain Responsiveness"; Arnér et al., "Lack of Analgesic Effect."

202 Merskey et al., *Classification of Chronic Pain.*

203 Meng et al., "Analgesia Circuit"; Rivers et al., "Development of Cannabinoid CBII Receptor Agonists."

204 Rivers et al., "Development of Cannabinoid CBII Receptor Agonists."

205 Rog et al., "Randomized Controlled Trial."

206 Wade et al., "Preliminary Controlled Study."

207 Berman et al., "Efficacy of Two Cannabis-Based Medicinal Extracts."

208 B. Wilsey, T. D. Marcotte, R. Deutsch, H. Zhao, H. Prasad, and A. Phan, "An Exploratory Human Laboratory Experiment Evaluating Vaporized Cannabis in the Treatment of Neuropathic Pain from Spinal Cord Injury and Disease," *Journal of Pain* 17:9 (2016), 982–1000.

209 Claudia Sommer, "Peripheral Neuropathies: Long-Term Opioid Therapy in Neuropathy: Benefit or Harm?" *Nature Reviews Neurology* 13 (2017), 516–17; N. B. Finnerup, N. Attal, S. Haroutounian, et al., "Pharmacotherapy for Neuropathic Pain in Adults: Systematic Review, Meta-Analysis and Updated NeuPSIG Recommendations," *The Lancet Neurology* 14:2 (2015), 162–73; E. M. Hoffman, J. C. Watson, J. St. Sauver, N. P. Staff, and C. J. Klein, "Association of Long-Term Opioid Therapy With Functional Status, Adverse Outcomes, and Mortality Among Patients With Polyneuropathy," *JAMA Neurol.* 74:7 (July 1, 2017), 773–79.

210 Sumner H. Burstein and Robert B. Zurier, "Cannabinoids, Endocannabinoids, and Related Analogs in Inflammation," *AAPS J.* 11:1 (March 2009), 109–19; B. Wilsey, T. Marcotte, A. Tsodikov, J. Millman, H. Bentley, B. Gouaux, and S. Fishman, "A Randomized, Placebo-Controlled, Crossover Trial of Cannabis Cigarettes in Neuropathic Pain," *J. Pain* 9:6 (June 2008), 506–21; N. Attal, L. Brasseur, D. Guirimand, S. Clermond-Gnamien, S. Atlami, and D. Bouhassira, "Are Oral Cannabinoids Safe and Effective in Refractory Neuropathic Pain?" *Eur. J. Pain* 8:2 (April 2004), 173–77; Berman et al., "Efficacy of Two Cannabis-Based Medicinal Extracts"; Wade et al., "Preliminary Controlled Study"; M. Karst, K. Salim, S. Burstein, I. Conrad, L. Hoy, and U. Schneider, "Analgesic Effect of the Synthetic Cannabinoid CT-3 on Chronic Neuropathic Pain: A Randomized Controlled Trial," *JAMA* 290:13 (October 1, 2003), 1757–62; T. J. Nurmikko, M. G. Serpell, B. Hoggart, et al., "Sativex Successfully Treats Neuropathic Pain Characterised by Allodynia: A Randomised, Doubleblind, Placebo-Controlled Clinical Trial," *Pain* 133 (2007), 210–20; William P.

Farquhar-Smith, "Peripheral Cannabinoid Analgesia: Neuronal and Immune Mechanisms," *Reviews in Analgesia* 8:2 (2005), 103–16; A. Ulugol, H. C. Karadag, Y. Ipci, M. Tamer, and I. Dokmeci, "The Effect of WIN 55,212-2, a Cannabinoid Agonist, on Tactile Allodynia in Diabetic Rats," *Neurosci. Lett.* 371:2–3 (November 23, 2004), 167–70; George W. Booz, "Cannabidiol as an Emergent Therapeutic Strategy for Lessening the Impact of Inflammation on Oxidative Stress," *Free Radic. Biol. Med.* 51:5 (September 1, 2011), 1054–61; M. S. Wallace, T. D. Marcotte, A. Umlauf, B. Gouaux, and J. H. Atkinson, "Efficacy of Inhaled Cannabis on Painful Diabetic Neuropathy," *J. Pain* 16:7 (July 2015), 616–27; D. I. Abrams, C. A. Jay, S. B. Shade, H. Vizoso, H. Reda, S. Press, M. E. Kelly, et al., "Cannabis in Painful HIV-Associated Sensory Neuropathy: A Randomized Placebo-Controlled Trial," *Neurology* 68:7 (February 13, 2007), 515–21; R. J. Ellis, W. Topero, F. Vaida, G. van den Brande, J. Gonzales, B. Gouaux, H. Bentley, and J. H. Atkinson, "Smoked Medicinal Cannabis for Neuropathic Pain in HIV: A Randomized, Crossover Clinical Trial," *Neuropsychopharmacology* 34:3 (February 2009), 672–80.

211 Sommer, "Peripheral Neuropathies."

212 Finnerup et al., "Pharmacotherapy for Neuropathic Pain."

213 Hoffman et al., "Association of Long-Term Opioid Therapy."

214 Burstein et al., "Cannabinoids, Endocannabinoids"; Attal et al., "Are Oral Cannabinoids Safe"; Berman et al., "Efficacy of Two Cannabis-Based Medicinal Extracts"; Wade et al., "Preliminary Controlled Study"; Karst et al., "Analgesic Effect"; Nurmikko et al., "Sativex Successfully Treats Neuropathic Pain"; Farquhar-Smith, "Peripheral Cannabinoid Analgesia."

215 Ulugol et al., "Effect of WIN 55,212-2"; Booz, "Cannabidiol as an Emergent Therapeutic Strategy"; Wallace et al., "Efficacy of Inhaled Cannabis."

216 Abrams et al., "Cannabis in Painful HIV-Associated Sensory Neuropathy"; Ellis et al., "Smoked medicinal cannabis."

217 L. Luongo, K. Starowicz, S. Maione, and V. Di Marzo, "Allodynia Lowering Induced by Cannabinoids and Endocannabinoids (ALICE)," *Pharmacol. Res.* 119 (May 2017), 272–77.

218 Barth Wilsey, Thomas D. Marcotte, Reena Deutsch, Ben Gouaux, Staci Sakai, and Haylee Donaghe, "Low Dose Vaporized Cannabis Significantly Improves Neuropathic Pain," *J. Pain* 14:2 (February 2013), 136–48.

219 F. Petzke, E. K. Enax-Krumova, and W. Häuser, "Efficacy, Tolerability and Safety of Cannabinoids for Chronic Neuropathic Pain: A Systematic Review of Randomized Controlled Studies. *Schmerz.* 30:1 (February 2016), 62–88.

220 C. Stein, "Targeting Pain and Inflammation by Peripherally Acting Opioids," *Frontiers in Pharmacology* 4 (2013), 123; E. Kalso, L. Smith, H. J. McQuay, R. A. Moore, "No Pain, No Gain: Clinical Excellence and Scientific Rigour—Lessons Learned from IA Morphine," *Pain* 98 (2002), 269–75; H. Gaskell, S. Derry, R. A. Moore, H. J. McQuay, "Single-Dose Oral Oxycodone and Oxycodone Plus Paracetamol (Acetaminophen) for Acute Postoperative Pain in Adults," *Cochrane Database Syst. Rev.* 2009:3, CD002763.

221 A. J. Stevens and M. D. Higgins, "A Systematic Review of the Analgesic Efficacy of Cannabinoid Medications in the Management of Acute Pain," *Acta Anaesthesiol. Scand.* 61:3 (March 2017), 268–80; K. Genaro, D. Fabris, A. L. F. Arantes, A. W. Zuardi, J. A. S. Crippa, and W. A. Prado, "Cannabidiol Is a Potential Therapeutic for the Affective-Motivational Dimension of Incision Pain in Rats," *Frontiers in Pharmacology* 8 (2017), 391; S. C. Britch, J. L. Wiley, Z. Yu, B. H. Clowers, and R. M. Craft, "Cannabidiol-Δ9-Tetrahydrocannabinol Interactions on Acute Pain and Locomotor Activity," *Drug Alcohol Depend.* 175 (June 1, 2017), 187–97; D. Raft, J. Gregg, J. Ghia, and L. Harris, "Effects of Intravenous Tetrahydrocannabinol on Experimental and Surgical Pain: Psychological Correlates of the Analgesic Response," *Clin. Pharmacol. Ther.* 21 (1977), 26–33.

222 Stein, "Targeting Pain"; Kalso et al., "No Pain, No Gain"; Gaskell et al., "Single Dose Oral Oxycodone."

223 Stevens et al., "Systematic Review of the Analgesic Efficacy"; Genaro et al., "Cannabidiol Is a Potential Therapeutic"; Britch et al., "Cannabidiol-Δ9-Tetrahydrocannabinol Interactions"; Raft et al., "Effects of Intravenous Tetrahydrocannabinol."

224 Genaro et al., "Cannabidiol Is a Potential Therapeutic."

225 Britch et al., "Cannabidiol-Δ9-Tetrahydrocannabinol Interactions."

226 Raft et al., "Effects of Intravenous Tetrahydrocannabinol."

227 J. C. Ballantyne and J. Mao, "Opioid Therapy for Chronic Pain," *N. Engl. J. Med.* 349 (2003), 1943–53; R. Chou, J. C. Ballantyne, G. J. Fanciullo, et al., "Research Gaps on Use of Opioids for Chronic Noncancer Pain: Findings from a Review of the Evidence for an American Pain Society and American Academy of Pain Medicine Clinical Practice Guideline," *J. Pain* 10 (2009), 147–59; J. C. Ballantyne, "Opioid Analgesia: Perspectives on Right Use and Utility," *Pain Physician* 10 (2007), 479–91.

228 Notcutt et al., "Initial experiences with medicinal extracts"; A. Dyson, M. Peacock, A. Chen, J. P. Courade, M. Yaqoob, A. Groarke, C. Brain, et al., "Antihyperalgesic Properties of the Cannabinoid CT-3 in Chronic Neuropathic and Inflammatory Pain States in the Rat," *Pain* 116:1–2 (July 2005), 129–37; Karst et al., "Analgesic Effect of the Synthetic Cannabinoid CT-3"; Ware et al., "Cannabis for the Management of Pain."

229 Ballantyne et al., "Opioid Therapy"; Chou et al., "Research Gaps"; Ballantyne, "Opioid analgesia."

230 Notcutt et al., "Initial Experiences with Medicinal Extracts."

231 Dyson et al., "Antihyperalgesic Properties of the Cannabinoid CT-3."

232 Karst et al., "Analgesic Effect of the Synthetic Cannabinoid CT-3."

233 Ware, et al., "Cannabis for the Management of Pain."

234 Adam Orens, Miles Light, Jacob Rowberry, Jeremy Matsen, and Brian Lewandowski, "Marijuana Equivalency in Portion and Dosage: An assessment of physical and pharmacokinetic relationships in marijuana production and consumption in Colorado," Colorado Department of Revenue, August 10, 2015.

235 Sumariwalla et al., "Novel Synthetic, Nonpsychoactive Cannabinoid Acid"; Costa et al., "Nonpsychoactive Cannabis Constituent Cannabidiol."

236 C. J. Woolf, "What Is This Thing Called Pain?" *Journal of Clinical Investigation* 120:11 (2010), 3742–44.

237 Gaskell et al., "Single-Dose Oral Oxycodone."

238 R. Schaefert, P. Welsch, P. Klose, C. Sommer, F. Petzke, and W. Häuser, "Opioids in Chronic Osteoarthritis Pain: A Systematic Review and Meta-analysis of Efficacy, Tolerability and Safety in Randomized Placebo-Controlled Studies of at Least 4 Weeks Duration," *Schmerz.* 29:1 (February 2015), 47–59.

239 A. Conte, C. M. Bettolo, E. Onesti, V. Frasca, E. Iacovelli, F. Gilio, E. Giacomelli, et al., "Cannabinoid-Induced Effects on the Nociceptive System: A Neurophysiological Study in Patients with Secondary Progressive Multiple Sclerosis," *Eur. J. Pain* 13:5 (May 2009), 472–77; D. Richardson, R. G. Pearson, N. Kurian, et al., "Characterisation of the Cannabinoid Receptor System in Synovial Tissue and Fluid in Patients with Osteoarthritis and Rheumatoid Arthritis," *Arthritis Res. Ther.* 10 (2008), R43; A. G. Hohmann and J. M. Walker, "Cannabinoid Suppression of Noxious Heat-Evoked Activity in Wide Dynamic Range Neuron in the Lumbar Dorsal Horn of the Rat," *J. Neurophysiol.* 81 (1999), 575–83; A. Dogrul, M. Seyrek, B. Yalcin, and A. Ulugol, "Involvement of Descending Serotonergic and Noradrenergic Pathways in CB1 Receptor-Mediated Antinociception," *Prog. Neuropsychopharmacol. Biol. Psychiatry* 38 (2012), 97–105.

240 Gaskell et al., "Single-Dose Oral Oxycodone."

241 Schaefert et al., "Opioids in Chronic Osteoarthritis Pain."

242 Conte et al., "Cannabinoid-Induced Effects on the Nociceptive System."

243 Richardson et al., "Characterisation of the Cannabinoid Receptor System."

244 Hohmann et al., "Cannabinoid Suppression."

245 Dogrul et al., "Involvement of Descending Serotonergic and Noradrenergic Pathways."

246 G. Watterson, R. Howard, and A. Goldman, "Peripheral Opioids in Inflammatory Pain," *Archives of Disease in Childhood* 89:7 (2004), 679–81.

247 Dai Lu, V. Kiran Vemuri, Richard I. Duclos Jr., and Alexandros Makriyannis, "The Cannabinergic System as a Target for Anti-Inflammatory Therapies," *Current Topics in Medicinal Chemistry* 6:13 (July 2006), 1401–26; Burstein et al., "Cannabinoids, endocannabinoids"; T. W. Klein, "Cannabinoid-Based Drugs as Anti-Inflammatory Therapeutics," *Nat. Rev. Immunol.* 5:5 (May 2005), 400–11; Sumner Burstein, "Ajulemic Acid (IP-751): Synthesis, Proof of Principle, Toxicity Studies, and Clinical Trials," *AAPS J.* 7:1 (March 2005), E143–48; J. Gertsch, M. Leonti, S. Raduner, et al., "Beta-Caryophyllene Is a Dietary Cannabinoid," *Proceedings of the National Academy of Sciences of the USA* 105:26 (2008), 9099–104; Booz, "Cannabidiol as an Emergent Therapeutic Strategy"; D. Katz, I. Katz, B. S. Porat-Katz, and Y. Shoenfeld, "Medical Cannabis: Another Piece in the Mosaic of Autoimmunity?" *Clin. Pharmacol. Ther.* 101:2 (February 2017), 230–38.

248 Watterson et al., "Peripheral Opioids."

249 S. Melik Parsadaniantz, C. Rivat, W. Rostene, and A. Reaux-Le Goazigo, "Opioid and Chemokine Receptor Crosstalk: A Promising Target for Pain Therapy?" *Nat. Rev. Neurosci.* 16 (2015), 69–78; N. M. Wilson, H. Jung, M. S. Ripsch, R. J. Miller, and F. A. White, "CXCR4 Signaling Mediates Morphine-Induced Tactile Hyperalgesia," *Brain Behav. Immun.* 25 (2011), 565–73; I. N. Johnston, E. D. Milligan, J. Wieseler-Frank, M. G. Frank, V. Zapata, J. Campisi, S. Langer, et al., "A Role for Proinflammatory Cytokines and Fractalkine in Analgesia, Tolerance, and Subsequent Pain Facilitation Induced by Chronic Intrathecal Morphine," *J. Neurosci.* 24 (2004), 7353–65.

250 I. A. Dhalla, T. Gomes, M. M. Mamdani, and D. N. Juurlink, "Opioids versus Nonsteroidal Anti-Inflammatory Drugs in NonCancer Pain," *Canadian Family Physician* 58:1 (2012), 30; World Health Organization, "WHO's Pain Ladder," 2011, www.who.int/cancer/palliative /painladder/en.

251 Lu et al., "Cannabinergic System."

252 Burstein et al., "Cannabinoids, Endocannabinoids."

253 Lu et al., "Cannabinergic System"; Klein, "Cannabinoid-Based Drugs"; Burstein, "Ajulemic Acid"; Gertsch et al., "Beta-Caryophyllene"; Booz, "Cannabidiol as an Emergent Therapeutic Strategy."

254 Katz et al., "Medical Cannabis."

255 Malfait et al., "Nonpsychoactive Cannabis Constituent Cannabidiol"; Wendy Swift, Peter Gates, and Paul Dillon, "Survey of Australians Using Cannabis for Medical Purposes," *Harm Reduct. J.* 2 (2005), 18.

256 S. Takeda, N. Usami, I. Yamamoto, and K. Watanabe, "Cannabidiol-2',6'-Dimethyl Ether, a Cannabidiol Derivative, Is a Highly Potent and Selective 15 Lipoxygenase Inhibitor," *Drug Metab. Dispos.* 37:8 (August 2009), 1733–37; Y. Zhao, Z. Yuan, Y. Liu, J. Xue, Y. Tian, W. Liu, W. Zhang, et. al., "Activation of Cannabinoid CB2 Receptor Ameliorates Atherosclerosis Associated with Suppression of Adhesion Molecules," *J. Cardiovasc. Pharmacol.* 9 (January 2010); M. Lanuti, E. Talamonti, M. Maccarrone, V. Chiurchiù, "Activation of GPR55 Receptors Exacerbates oxLDL-Induced Lipid Accumulation and Inflammatory Responses, while Reducing Cholesterol Efflux from Human Macrophages," *PLoS ONE* 10:5 (2015), e0126839; Z. Zhang, C. Yang, X. Dai, Y. Ao, and Y. Li, "Inhibitory Effect of Trans-Caryophyllene (TC) on Leukocyte-Endothelial Attachment," *Toxicol. Appl. Pharmacol.* 329 (June 15, 2017), 326–33.

257 H. Krenn, L. K. Daha, W. Oczenski, and R. D. Fitzgerald, "A Case of Cannabinoid Rotation in a Young Woman with Chronic Cystitis," *J. Pain Symptom Manag.* 25:1 (January 2003), 3–4.

258 D. R. Blake, P. Robson, M. Ho, R. W. Jubb, and C. S. McCabe, "Preliminary Assessment of the Efficacy, Tolerability and Safety of a Cannabis-Based Medicine (Sativex) in the Treatment of Pain Caused by Rheumatoid Arthritis," *Rheumatology* 45:1 (2006), 50–52; J. Parker, F.

Atez, R. G. Rossetti, A. Skulas, R. Patel, and R. B. Zurier, "Suppression of Human Macrophage Interleukin-6 by a Nonpsychoactive Cannabinoid Acid," *Rheumatol. Int.* 28:7 (May 2008), 631–35.

259 H. Beaumont, J. Jensen, A. Carlsson, M. Ruth, A. Lehmann, and G. E. Boeckx-staens, "Effect of Delta(9)-Tetrahydrocannabinol, a Cannabinoid Receptor Agonist, on the Triggering of Transient Lower Esoesophageal Sphincter Relaxations in Dogs and Humans," *Br. J. Pharmacol.* 156:1 (January 2009), 153–62; Y. Tambe, H. Tsujiuchi, G. Honda, Y. Ikeshiro, and S. Tanaka, "Gastric Cytoprotection of the nonSteroidal Anti-inflammatory Sesquiterpene, Beta-Caryophyllene," *Planta Med.* 62:5 (October 1996), 469–70; Omar Abdel-Salam, "Gastric Acid Inhibitory and Gastric Protective Effects of Cannabis and Cannabinoids," *Asian Pacific Journal of Tropical Medicine* 9:5 (May 2016), 413–19.

260 M. A. Storr, C. M. Keenan, D. Emmerdinger, H. Zhang, B. Yüce, A. Sibaev, F. Massa, et al., "Targeting Endocannabinoid Degradation Protects against Experimental Colitis in Mice: Involvement of CB(1) and CB(2) Receptors," *J. Mol. Med.* (Berl.) 86:8 (August 2008), 925–36; R. Capasso, F. Borrelli, G. Aviello, B. Romano, C. Scalisi, F. Capasso, and A. Izzo, "Cannabidiol, Extracted from *Cannabis sativa,* Selectively Inhibits in Ammatory Hypermotility in Mice," *Br. J. Pharmacol.* 154:5 (July 2008), 1001–08; F. Borrelli, G. Aviello, B. Romano, P. Orlando, R. Capasso, F. Maiello, F. Guadagno, et al., "Cannabidiol, a Safe and Non-Psychotropic Ingredient of the Marijuana Plant *Cannabis sativa,* Is Protective in a Murine Model Of Colitis," *J. Mol. Med.* (Berl.) 87:11 (November 2009), 1111–21; A. F. Bento, R. Marcon, R. C. Dutra, et al., "⊠-Caryophyllene Inhibits Dextran Sulfate Sodium-Induced Colitis in Mice through CB2 Receptor Activation and PPAR⊠ Pathway," *American Journal of Pathology*178:3 (2011), 1153–66; U. P. Phatak, D. Rojas-Velasquez, A. Porto, and D. S. Pashankar, "Prevalence and Patterns of Marijuana Use in Young Adults with Inflammatory Bowel Disease," *J. Pediatr. Gastroenterol. Nutr.* 64:2 (February 2017), 261–64; E. Pagano, R. Capasso, F. Piscitelli, B. Romano, O. A. Parisi, S. Finizio, A. Lauritano, et al., "An Orally Active Cannabis Extract with High Content in Cannabidiol attenuates Chemically-Induced Intestinal Inflammation and Hypermotility in the Mouse," *Front. Pharmacol.* 4:7 (October 2016), 341; H. Shamran, N. P. Singh, E. E. Zumbrun, A. Murphy, D. D. Taub, M. K. Mishra, R. L. Price, et al., "Fatty Acid Amide Hydrolase (FAAH) Blockade Ameliorates Experimental Colitis by Altering MicroRNA Expression and Suppressing Inflammation," *Brain Behav. Immun.* 59 (January 2017), 10–20.

261 Christoph W. Michalski, Milena Maier, Mert Erkan, Danguole Sauliunaite, Frank Bergmann, Pal Pacher, Sandor Batkai, et al., "Cannabinoids Reduce Markers of Inflammation and Fibrosis in Pancreatic Stellate Cells," *PLoS ONE* 3:2 (2008), e1701; A. Dembiński, Z. Warzecha, P. Ceranowicz, A. M. Warzecha, W. W. Pawlik, M. Dembiński, K. Rembiasz, et al., "Dual, Time-Dependent Deleterious and Protective Effect of Anandamide on the Course of Cerulein-Induced Acute Pancreatitis: Role of Sensory Nerves," *Eur. J. Pharmacol.* 591:1–3 (September 4, 2008), 284–92; K. Matsuda, Y. Mikami, K. Takeda, S. Fukuyama,

S. Egawa, M. Sunamura, I. Maruyama, and S. Matsuno, "The Cannabinoid 1 Receptor Antagonist, AM251, Prolongs the Survival of Rats with Severe Acute Pancreatitis," *Tohoku J. Exp. Med.* 207:2 (October 2005), 99–107; W. K. Utomo, M. de Vries, H. Braat, et al., "Modulation of Human Peripheral Blood Mononuclear Cell Signaling by Medicinal Cannabinoids," *Frontiers in Molecular Neuroscience* 10 (2017), 14.

262 M. H. Napimoga, B. B. Benatti, F. O. Lima, P. M. Alves, A. C. Campos, D. R. Pena-Dos-Santos, F. P. Severino, F. Q. Cunha, and F. S. Guimarães, "Cannabidiol Decreases Bone Resorption by Inhibiting RANK/RANKL Expression and Pro-inflammatory Cytokines During Experimental Periodontitis in Rats," *Int. Immunopharmacol.* 9:2 (February 2009), 216–22.

263 J. Mao, D. D. Price, J. Lu, L. Keniston, and D. J. Mayer, "Two Distinctive Antinociceptive Systems in Rats with Pathological Pain," *Neurosci. Lett.* 280:1 (February 11, 2000), 13–6.

264 Ibid.

265 Woolf, "What Is This Thing Called Pain?"

266 Jenny L. Wilkerson and Erin D. Milligan, "The Central Role of Glia in Pathological Pain and the Potential of Targeting the Cannabinoid 2 Receptor for Pain Relief," *ISRN Anesthesiology* 2011 (2011), article ID 593894.

267 Mao et al., "Two Distinctive Antinociceptive Systems."

268 R. A. Slivicki, Z. Xu, P. M. Kulkarni, R. G. Pertwee, K. Mackie, G. A. Thakur, and A. G. Hohmann, "Positive Allosteric Modulation of Cannabinoid Receptor Type 1 Suppresses Pathological Pain Without Producing Tolerance or Dependence," *Biol. Psychiatry* pii: S0006-3223:17 (July 8, 2017), 31761–64.

269 Ibid.

270 American Psychiatric Association, *DSM-5.*

271 *Odyssey,* book 4, v. 219–21.

272 E. J. Khantzian, "The Self-Medication Hypothesis of Addictive Disorders: Focus on Heroin and Cocaine Dependence," *American Journal of Psychiatry* 142:11 (1985), 1259–64.

273 B. J. Piper, R. M. DeKeuster, M. L. Beals, C. M. Cobb, C. A. Burchman, L. Perkinson, S. T. Lynn, et al., "Substitution of Medical Cannabis for Pharmaceutical Agents for Pain, Anxiety, and Sleep," *J. Psychopharmacol.* 31:5 (May 2017), 569–75; J. M. Corroon Jr., L. K. Mischley, and M. Sexton, "Cannabis as a Substitute for Prescription Drugs: A Cross-sectional Study," *J. Pain. Res.* 10 (May 2, 2017), 989–98.

274 M. Fujimori and H. E. Himwich, "Delta 9-Tetrahydrocannabinol and the Sleep-Wakefulness Cycle in Rabbits," *Physiol. Behav.* 11:3 (September 1973), 291–95; I. Feinberg, R. Jones, J. M. Walker, C. Cavness, and J. March, "Effects of High Dosage Delta-9-Tetrahydrocannabinol on Sleep Patterns in Man," *Clin. Pharmacol. Ther.* 17:4 (April 1975), 458–66; P. M. Adams and E. S. Barratt, "Effect of Chronic Marijuana Administration of Stages of Primate Sleep-Wakefulness," *Biol. Psychiatry* 10:3 (June 1975), 315–22; I. Feinberg, R. Jones, J. M. Walker, C. Cavness, and T. Floyd, "Effects of Marijuana Extract and Tetrahydrocannabinol

on Electroencephalographic Sleep Patterns," *Clin. Pharmacol. Ther.* 19:6 (June 1976), 782–94; Jaime M. Monti, "Hypnoticlike Effects of Cannabidiol in the Rat," *Psychopharmacology* 55:3 (January 1977) 263–65; E. A. Carlini and J. M. Cunha, "Hypnotic and Antiepileptic Effects of Cannabidiol," *J. Clin. Pharmacol.* 21:8–9 suppl. (August–September 1981), 417S–427S; E. Murillo-Rodríguez, M. Sánchez-Alavez, L. Navarro, D. Martínez-González, R. Drucker-Colín, and O. Prospéro-García, "Anandamide Modulates Sleep and Memory in Rats," *Brain Res.* 812:1–2 (November 23, 1998), 270–74; Anthony N. Nicholson, Claire Turner, Barbara M. Stone, and Philip J. Robson, "Effect of D-9-Tetrahydrocannabinol and Cannabidiol on Nocturnal Sleep and Early-Morning Behavior in Young Adults," *Journal of Clinical Psychopharmacology* 24:3 (June 2004); Swift et al., "Survey of Australians"; Eric Murillo-Rodríguez, Andrea Sarro-Ramírez, Daniel Sánchez, Stephanie Mijangos-Moreno, Alma Tejeda-Padrón, Alwin Poot-Aké, Khalil Guzmán, et al., "Potential Effects of Cannabidiol as a Wake-Promoting Agent," *Curr. Neuropharmacol.* 12:3 (May 2014), 269–72; S. Shannon and J. Opila-Lehman, "Effectiveness of Cannabidiol Oil for Pediatric Anxiety and Insomnia as Part of Posttraumatic Stress Disorder: A Case Report," *Perm. J.* 20:4 (Fall 2016), 108–11; David A. Gorelick, Robert S. Goodwin, Eugene Schwilke, Jennifer R. Schroeder, David M. Schwope, Deanna L. Kelly, Catherine Ortemann-Renon, et al., "Around-the-Clock Oral THC Effects on Sleep in Male Chronic Daily Cannabis Smokers," *American Journal on Addiction* 22:5 (September–October 2013), 510–14; Rolando Tringale and Claudia Jensen, "Cannabis and Insomnia," *O'Shaughnessy's* Autumn 2011, 31–32; J. A. Crippa, A. W. Zuardi, R. Martín-Santos, S. Bhattacharyya, Z. Atakan, P. McGuire, and P. Fusar-Poli, "Cannabis and Anxiety: A Critical Review of the Evidence," *Hum. Psychopharmacol.* 24:7 (October 2009), 515–23; Noriyuki Usami, Takeshi Okuda, Hisatoshi Yoshida, Toshiyuki Kimura, Kazuhito Watanabe, Hidetoshi Yoshimura, and Ikuo Yamamoto, "Synthesis and Pharmacological Evaluation in Mice of Halogenated Cannabidiol Derivatives," *Chem. Pharm. Bull.* 47:11 (1999), 1641–45; R. N. Takahashi and I. G. Karniol, "Pharmacologic Interaction between Cannabinol and Delta-9-Tetrahydrocannabinol," *Psychopharmacologia* 41:3 (1975), 277–84; D. R. Keith, E. W. Gunderson, M. Haney, R. W. Foltin, and C. L. Hart, "Smoked Marijuana Attenuates Performance and Mood Disruptions During Simulated Night Shift Work," *Drug Alcohol Depend.* 178 (September 1, 2017), 534–43; Piper et al., "Substitution of Medical Cannabis."

275 J. E. Beal, R. Olson, L. Laubenstein, J. O. Morales, P. Bellman, B. Yangco, L. Lefkowitz, et al., "Dronabinol as a Treatment for Anorexia Associated with Weight Loss in Patients with AIDS," *Journal of Pain and Symptom Management* 10:2 (1995), 89–97; G. W. Neff, C. B. O'Brien, K. R. Reddy, N. V. Bergasa, A. Regev, E. Molina, R. Amaro, et al., "Preliminary Observation with Dronabinol in Patients with Intractable Pruritus Secondary to Cholestatic Liver Disease," *Am. J. Gastroenterol.* 97:8 (August 2002), 2117–19; Wen Jiang, Yun Zhang, Lan Xiao, Jamie Van Cleemput, Shao-Ping Ji, Guang Bai, and Xia Zhang, "Cannabinoids Promote Embryonic and Adult Hippocampus Neurogenesis and Produce Anxiolytic- and

Antidepressant-like Effects," *J. Clin. Invest.* 115:11 (2005), 3104–16; R. J. McLaughlin, M. N. Hill, A. C. Morrish, and B. B. Gorzalka, "Local Enhancement of Cannabinoid CB1 Receptor Signaling in the Dorsal Hippocampus Elicits an Antidepressant-like Effect," *Behav. Pharmacol.* 18:5–6 (September 2007), 431–38; F. R. Bambico, N. Katz, G. Debonnel, and G. Gobbi, "Cannabinoids Elicit Antidepressant-like Behavior and Activate Serotonergic Neurons through the Medial Prefrontal Cortex," *J. Neurosci.* 27:43 (2007), 11700–11; I. B. Corless, T. Lindgren, W. Holzemer, L. Robinson, S. Moezzi, K. Kirksey, C. Coleman, et al., "Marijuana Effectiveness as an HIV Self-Care Strategy," *Clin. Nurs. Res.* 18:2 (May 2009), 172–93; Crippa et al., "Therapeutical Use"; Abir T. El-Alfy, Kelly Ivey, Keisha Robinson, Safwat Ahmed, Mohamed Radwan, Desmond Slade, Ikhlas Khan, et al., "Antidepressant-like Effect of Δ9-Tetrahydrocannabinol and Other Cannabinoids Isolated from *Cannabis sativa* L.," *Pharmacology Biochemistry and Behavior* 95:4 (June 2010), 434–42; Booz, "Cannabidiol as an Emergent Therapeutic Strategy"; Alline Cristina Campos, Fabricio Araújo Moreira, Felipe Villela Gomes, Elaine Aparecida Del Bel, and Francisco Silveira Guimarães, "Multiple Mechanisms Involved in the Large-Spectrum Therapeutic Potential of Cannabidiol in Psychiatric Disorders," *Philos. Trans. R. Soc. Lond. B Biol. Sci.* 367:1607 (December 5, 2012); F. R. Bambico, P. R. Hattan, J. P. Garant, and G. Gobbi, "Effect of Delta-9-Tetrahydrocannabinol on Behavioral Despair and on Pre- and Postsynaptic Serotonergic Transmission," *Prog. Neuropsychopharmacol. Biol. Psychiatry* 38:1 (July 2, 2012), 88–96; A. Bahi, S. Mansouri, E. Memari, M. Ameri, S. M. Nurulain, and S. Ojha, "⊠-Caryophyllene, a CB2 Receptor Agonist Produces Multiple Behavioral Changes Relevant to Anxiety and Depression in Mice," *Physiol. Behav.* 135 (August 2014), 119–24; Gruber et al., "Splendor in the Grass?"; G. Shoval, L. Shbiro, L. Hershkovitz, N. Hazut, G. Zalsman, R. Mechoulam, and A. Weller, "Prohedonic Effect of Cannabidiol in a Rat Model of Depression," *Neuropsychobiology* 73:2 (2016),123–9; A. C. Campos, M. V. Fogaça, A. B. Sonego, and F. S. Guimarães, "Cannabidiol, Neuroprotection and Neuropsychiatric Disorders," *Pharmacol. Res.* 112 (October 2016), 119–27; Emily Boorman, Zuzanna Zajkowska, Rumsha Ahmed, Carmine M. Pariante, and Patricia A. Zunszain, "Crosstalk between Endocannabinoid and Immune Systems: A Potential Dysregulation in Depression?" *Psychopharmacology* (Berl). 233 (2016), 1591–1604; R. Linge, L. Jiménez-Sánchez, L. Campa, F. Pilar-Cuéllar, R. Vidal, A. Pazos, A. Adell, and Á. Díaz, "Cannabidiol Induces Rapid-Acting Antidepressant-like Effects and Enhances Cortical 5-HT/Glutamate Neurotransmission: Role of 5-HT1A Receptors," *Neuropharmacology* 103 (April 2016), 16-26; A. G. Sartim, F. S. Guimarães, and S. R. Joca, "Antidepressant-like Effect of Cannabidiol Injection into the Ventral Medial Prefrontal Cortex-Possible Involvement of 5-HT1A and CB1 Receptors," *Behav. Brain Res.* 303 (April 15, 2016), 218–27; Alline C. Campos, Manoela V. Fogaça, Franciele F. Scarante, Sâmia R. L. Joca, Amanda J. Sales, Felipe V. Gomes, Andreza B. Sonego, et al., "Plastic and Neuroprotective Mechanisms Involved in the Therapeutic Effects of Cannabidiol in Psychiatric Disorders," *Front. Pharmacol.* May 23, 2017; Corroon et al., "Cannabis as a Substitute";

Rebecca J. Bluett, Rita Báldi, Andre Haymer, Andrew D. Gaulden, Nolan D. Hartley, Walker P. Parrish, Jordan Baechle, et al., "Endocannabinoid Signalling Modulates Susceptibility to Traumatic Stress Exposure," *Nature Communications* 8, article no. 14782 (2017); El-Alfy et al., "Antidepressant-like Effect"; A. Zuardi, J. Crippa, S. Dursun, S. Morais, J. Vilela, R. Sanches, and J. Hal-lak, "Cannabidiol Was Ineffective for Manic Episode of Bipolar Affective Disorder," *J. Psychopharmacol.* 24:1 (January 2010), 135–37; R. S. El-Mallakh and C. Brown, "The Effect of Extreme Marijuana Use on the Long-Term Course of Bipolar I Illness: A Single Case Study," *J. Psychoactive Drugs* 39:2 (2007), 201–2; C. H. Ashton, P. B. Moore, P. Gallagher, and A. H. Young, "Cannabinoids in Bipolar Affective Disorder: A Review and Discussion of Their Therapeutic Potential," *J. Psychopharmacol.* 19:3 (May 2005), 293–300; L. Grinspoon and J. B. Bakalar, "The Use of Cannabis as a Mood Stabilizer in Bipolar Disorder: Anecdotal Evidence and the Need for Clinical Research," *J. Psychoactive Drugs* 30:2 (April–June 1998), 171–77.

276 Philip H. Smith, Gregory G. Homish, R. Lorraine Collins, Gary A. Giovino, Helene R. White, and Kenneth E. Leonard, "Couples' Marijuana Use Is Inversely Related to Their Intimate Partner Violence over the First Nine Years of Marriage," *Psychol. Addict. Behav.* 28:3 (September 2014), 734–42.

277 T. F. Plasse, R. W. Gorter, S. H. Krasnow, M. Lane, K. V. Shepard, and R. G. Wadleigh, "Recent Clinical Experience with Dronabinol," *Pharmacol. Biochem. Behav.* 40:3 (November 1991), 695–700; K. Nelson, D. Walsh, P. Deeter, and F. Sheehan, "A Phase II Study Of Delta-9-Tetrahydrocannabinol for Appetite Stimulation in Cancer-Associated Anorexia," *Journal of Palliative Care* 10:1 (1994), 14–18; Beal et al., "Dronabinol as a treatment"; R. Gómez, M. Navarro, B. Ferrer, J. M. Trigo, A. Bilbao, I. Del Arco, A. Cippitelli, et al., "A Peripheral Mechanism for CB1 Cannabinoid Receptor-Dependent Modulation of Feeding," *J. Neurosci.* 22:21 (November 1, 2002), 9612–17; T. C. Kirkham, "Endocannabinoids in the Regulation of Appetite and Body Weight," *Behav. Pharmacol.* 16:5–6 (September 2005), 297–313; Y. H. Jo, Y. J. Chen, S. C. Chua Jr., D. A. Talmage, and L. W. Role, "Integration of Endocannabinoid and Leptin Signaling in an Appetite-Related Neural Circuit," *Neuron* 48:6 (December 22, 2005), 1055–66; V. Maida, "The Synthetic Cannabinoid Nabilone Improves Pain and Symptom Management in Cancer Patients," paper presented at the San Antonio Breast Cancer Symposium, December 2006; F. Strasser, D. Luftner, K. Possinger, G. Ernst, T. Ruhstaller, W. Meissner, Y. D. Ko, et al., "Comparison of Orally Administered Cannabis Extract and Delta-9 Tetrahydrocannabinol in Treating Patients with Cancer-Related Anorexia-Cachexia Syndrome: A Multicenter, Phase III, Randomized, Double-Blind, Placebo-Controlled Clinical Trial from the Cannabis-in-Cachexia-Study-Group," *J. Clin. Oncol.* 24:21 (2006), 3394–3400; E. Dejesus, B. M. Rodwick, D. Bowers, C. J. Cohen, and D. Pearce, "Use of Dronabinol Improves Appetite and Reverses Weight Loss in HIV/ AIDS-Infected Patients," *J. Int. Assoc. Physicians AIDS Care* 6:2 (2007), 95–100; M. M. Wilson, C. Philpot, and J. E. Morley, "Anorexia of Aging in Long-Term

Care: Is Dronabinol an Effective Appetite Stimulant?—a Pilot Study," *J. Nutr. Health Aging* 11:2 (March–April 2007), 195–98; C. T. Costiniuk, E. Mills, and C. L. Cooper, "Evaluation of Oral Cannabinoid-Containing Medications for the Management of Interferon and Ribavirin-Induced Anorexia, Nausea and Weight Loss in Patients Treated for Chronic Hepatitis C Virus," *Can. J. Gastroenterol.* 22:4 (April 2008), 376–80; D. I. Brierley, J. Samuels, M. Duncan, B. J. Whalley, and C. M. Williams, "Cannabigerol Is a Novel, Well-Tolerated Appetite Stimulant in Pre-satiated Rats," *Psychopharmacology* 2016;233(19):3603-3613; Kaur et al., "Endocannabinoid System"; D. I. Brierley, J. Samuels, M. Duncan, B. J. Whalley, and C. M. Williams, "A Cannabigerol-Rich Cannabis Sativa Extract, Devoid of 9-Tetrahydrocannabinol, Elicits Hyperphagia in Rats," *Behav. Pharmacol.* 28:4 (June 2017), 280–84.

278 L. M. Shin, S. L. Rauch, and R. K. Pitman, "Amygdala, Medial Prefrontal Cortex, and Hippocampal Function in PTSD," *Ann. NY Acad. Sci.* 1071 (July 2006), 67–79.

279 L. K. Jacobsen, S. M. Southwick, and T. R. Kosten, "Substance Use Disorders in Patients with Posttraumatic Stress Disorder: A Review of the Literature," *American Journal of Psychiatry* 158 (2001), 1184–90.

280 D. A. Hien, H. Jiang, A. N. C. Campbell, M. C. Hu, G. M. Miele, L. R. Cohen, G. S. Brigham, et al., "Do Treatment Improvements in PTSD Severity Affect Substance Use Outcomes? A Secondary Analysis from a Randomized Clinical Trial in NIDA's Clinical Trials Network," *American Journal of Psychiatry* 167 (2010), 95–101.

281 Ibid.

282 Bethany Ketchen, Pamela Eilender, and Ayman Fareed, "Comorbid Post Traumatic Stress Disorder, Pain and Opiate Addiction," in Colin R. Martin, Victor R. Preedy, and Vinood B. Patel, *Comprehensive Guide to Post-Traumatic Stress Disorder* (New York: Springer, 2015), 1–21; K. T. Brady, P. Tuerk, S. E. Back, M. E. Saladin, A. E. Waldrop, H. Myrick, "Combat Posttraumatic Stress Disorder, Substance Use Disorders, and Traumatic Brain Injury," *Journal of Addiction Medicine* 3:4 (2009), 179–88.

283 J. L. McCauley, T. Killeen, D. F. Gros, K. T. Brady, S. E. Back, "Posttraumatic Stress Disorder and Co-Occurring Substance Use Disorders: Advances in Assessment and Treatment," *Clinical Psychology* 19:3 (2012), 283–304; L. B. Cottler, W. M. Compton III, D. Mager, E. L. Spitznagel, and A. Janca, "Posttraumatic Stress Disorder among Substance Users from the General Population," *Am. J. Psychiatry* 149:5 (May 1992), 664–70; Jacobsen et al., "Substance use disorders"; K. L. Mills, M. Teesson, J. Ross, and L. Peters, "Trauma, PTSD, and Substance Use Disorders: Findings from the Australian National Survey of Mental Health and Well-Being," *Am. J. Psychiatry* 163:4 (April 2006), 652–8; R. C. Kessler, "Posttraumatic Stress Disorder: The Burden to the Individual and to Society," *J. Clin. Psychiatry* 61 (2000) suppl. 5, 4–12, discussion 13.4; J. D. Bremner, S. M Southwick, A. Darnell, and D. S. Charney, "Chronic PTSD in Vietnam Combat Veterans: Course of Illness and Substance Abuse," *Am. J. Psychiatry* 153:3 (March 1996), 369–75.

284 A. Fareed, P. Eilender, M. Haber, J. Bremner, N. Whitfield, and K. Drexler, "Comorbid Posttraumatic Stress Disorder and Opiate Addiction: A Literature Review," *J. Addict. Dis.* 32:2 (2013), 168–79.

285 D. van Dam, E. Vedel, T. Ehring, and P. M. G. Emmelkamp, "Psychological Treatments for Concurrent Posttraumatic Stress Disorder and Substance Use Disorder: A Systematic Review," *Clinical Psychology Review* 32 (2012), 202–14; Institute of Medicine, Committee on Treatment of Posttraumatic Stress, *Treatment of Posttraumatic Stress Disorder: An Assessment of the Evidence* (Washington, DC: National Academies Press, 2008); Ketchen et al., "Comorbid Post Traumatic Stress Disorder."

286 J. Shurman, G. F. Koob, and H. B. Gutstein, "Opioids, Pain, the Brain, and Hyperkatifeia: A Framework for the Rational Use of Opioids for Pain," *Pain Medicine* 11:7 (2010), 1092–98.

287 Luongo et al., "Allodynia Lowering."

288 L. M. Dufton, B. Konik, R. Colletti, C. Stanger, M. Boyer, S. Morrow, B. E. Compas, "Effects of Stress on Pain Threshold and Tolerance in Children with Recurrent Abdominal Pain," *Pain* 136:1–2 (2008), 38–43; L. Quintero, M. Moreno, C. Avila, J. Arcaya, W. Maixner, and H. Suarez-Roca, "Long-lasting Delayed Hyperalgesia after Subchronic Swim Stress," *Pharmacol. Biochem. Behav.* 67:3 (2000), 449–58; I. L. da Silva Torres, S. N. Cucco, M. Bassani, M. S. Duarte, P. P. Silveira, A. P. Vasconcellos, A. S. Tabajara, et al., "Long-lasting Delayed Hyperalgesia after Chronic Restraint Stress in Rats: Effect Of Morphine Administration," *Neurosci. Res.* 45:3 (2003), 277–83; C. Tsigos and G. P. Chrousos, "Hypothalamic-Pituitary-Adrenal Axis, Neuroendocrine Factors and Stress," *J. Psychosom. Res.* 53:4 (October 2002), 865–71.

289 E. M. Jennings, B. N. Okine, M. Roche, and D. P. Finn, "Stress-Induced Hyperalgesia," *Prog. Neurobiol.* 121 (2014), 1–18.

290 T. M. Palermo, E. F. Law, J Fales, M. H. Bromberg, T. Jessen-Fiddick, G. Tai, "Internet-Delivered Cognitive-Behavioral Treatment for Adolescents with Chronic Pain and Their Parents: A Randomized Controlled Multicenter Trial, *Pain* 157:1 (2016), 174–85.

291 Kentucky Department for Public Health, Division of Maternal and Child Health, "Neonatal Abstinence Syndrome in Kentucky." Data brief, December 2015.

292 R. C. Frederickson, C. R. Hewes, and J. W. Aiken, "Correlation between the In Vivo and an In Vitro Expression of Opiate Withdrawal Precipitated by Naloxone: Their Antagonism by l-(-)-Delta9-Tetrahydrocannabinol," *J. Pharmacol. Exp. Ther.* 199:2 (November 1976), 375–84; G. Vela, M. Ruiz-Gayo, and J. A. Fuentes, "Anandamide Decreases Naloxone-Precipitated Withdrawal Signs in Mice Chronically Treated with Morphine," *Neuropharmacology* 34:6 (June 1995), 665–68; T. Rubino, P. Massi, D. Viganò, D. Fuzio, and D. Parolaro, "Long-Term Treatment with SR141716A, the CB1 Receptor Antagonist, Influences Morphine Withdrawal Syndrome," *Life Sci.* 66:22 (April 21, 2000), 2213–19; Magdalena Mas-Nieto, Blandine Pommier, Eleni T Tzavara, Anne Caneparo, Sophie Da Nascimento, Gérard

Le Fur, Bernard P Roques, and Florence Noble, "Reduction of Opioid Dependence by the CB1 Antagonist SR141716A in Mice: Evaluation of the Interest in Pharmacotherapy of Opioid Addiction," *Br. J. Pharmacol.* 132:8 (April 2001), 1809–16; McPartland et al., "Meta-analysis of Cannabinoid Ligand Binding Affinity"; K. A. Seely, L. K. Brents, L. N. Franks, M. Rajasekaran, S. M. Zimmerman, W. E. Fantegrossi, P. L. Prather, "AM-251 and Rimonabant Act as Direct Antagonists at Mu-Opioid Receptors: Implications for Opioid/Cannabinoid Interaction Studies." *Neuropharmacology* 63 (2012), 905–15; European Medicines Agency, "The European Medicines Agency Recommends Suspension of the Marketing Authorisation of Acomplia," October 23, 2008. Doc. ref. EMEA/CHMP/537777/2008; F. A. Moreira and J. A. Crippa, "The Psychiatric Side-Effects of Rimonabant," *Rev. Bras. Psiquiatr.* 31:2 (June 2009), 145–53; European Medicines Agency, "Medicinal Product No Longer Authorized: Acomplia (rimonabant)," January 30, 2009, http://goo.gl/yB6tu1; T. Yamaguchi, Y. Hagiwara, H. Tanaka, T. Sugiura, K. Waku, Y. Shoyama, S. Watanabe, and T. Yamamoto, "Endogenous Cannabinoid, 2-Arachidonoylglycerol, Attenuates Naloxone-Precipitated Withdrawal Signs in Morphine-Dependent Mice," *Brain Res.* 909:1–2 (August 3, 2001), 121–26; A. H. Lichtman, S. M. Sheikh, H. H. Loh, and B. R. Martin, "Opioid and Cannabinoid Modulation of Precipitated Withdrawal in Delta(9)-Tetrahydrocannabinol and Morphine-Dependent Mice," *J. Pharmacol. Exp. Ther.* 298:3 (September 2001), 1007–14; O. Valverde, F. Noble, F. Beslot, V. Daugé, M. C. Fournié-Zaluski, and B. P. Roques, "Delta9-Tetrahydrocannabinol Releases and Facilitates the Effects of Endogenous Enkephalins: Reduction in Morphine Withdrawal Syndrome without Change in Rewarding Effect," *Eur. J. Neurosci.* 13:9 (May 2001), 1816–24; I. Del Arco, M. Navarro, A. Bilbao, B. Ferrer, D. Piomelli, and F. Rodríguez De Fonseca, "Attenuation of Spontaneous Opiate Withdrawal in Mice by the Anandamide Transport Inhibitor AM404. *Eur. J. Pharmacol.* 454:1 (November 1, 2002), 103–4; D. L. Cichewicz and S. P. Welch, "Modulation of Oral Morphine Antinociceptive Tolerance and Naloxone-Precipitated Withdrawal Signs by Oral Delta 9-Tetrahydrocannabinol," *J. Pharmacol. Exp. Ther.* 305:3 (June 2003), 812–17; M. L. Cox, V. L. Haller, and S. P. Welch, "Synergy between Delta9-Tetrahydrocannabinol and Morphine in the Arthritic Rat," *Eur. J. Pharmacol.* 567:1–2 (July 12, 2007), 125–30; D. I. Abrams, P. Couey, S. B. Shade, M. E. Kelly, N. L. Benowitz, "Cannabinoid-Opioid Interaction in Chronic Pain," *Clin. Pharmacol. Ther.* 90:6 (December 2011), 844–51; M. Collen, "Prescribing Cannabis for Harm Reduction," *Harm Reduction Journal* 9 (2012), 1; G. T. Carter, A. M. Flanagan, M. Earleywine, D. I. Abrams, S. K. Aggarwal, and L. Grinspoon, "Cannabis in Palliative Medicine: Improving Care and Reducing Opioid-Related Morbidity," *Am. J. Hosp. Palliat. Care* 28 (2011), 297–303; J. L. Scavone, R. C. Sterling, E. J. Van Bockstaele, "Cannabinoid and Opioid Interactions: Implications for Opiate Dependence and Withdrawal," *Neuroscience* 248 (2013), 637–54; Bachhuber, "Medical Cannabis Laws"; Staci A. Gruber, Kelly A. Sagar, Mary K. Dahlgren, Megan T. Racine, Rosemary T. Smith, and Scott E. Lukas, "Splendor in the Grass? A Pilot Study Assessing the Impact of Medical

Marijuana on Executive Function," *Front. Pharmacol.* 7 (October 13, 2016), 355; George F. Koob, "The Dark Side of Emotion: The Addiction Perspective," *Eur. J. Pharmacol.* 753 (April 15, 2015), 73–87; Crippa et al., "Therapeutical Use"; F. M. Lewekel, D. Koethe, F. Pahlisch, D. Schreiber, C. W. Gerth, B. M. Nol-den, J. Klosterkötter, et al., "S39-02 Antipsychotic Effects of Cannabidiol," *European Psychiatry* 24 (2009), suppl. 1, S207; J. Fernández-Ruiz, O. Sagredo, M. R. Pazos, et al., "Cannabidiol for Neurodegenerative Disorders: Important New Clinical Applications for This Phytocannabinoid?" *British Journal of Clinical Pharmacology* 75:2 (2013), 323–33; Iuvone et al., "Cannabidiol"; A. Pelliccia, G. Grassi, A. Romano, and P. Crocchialo, "Treatment with CBD in Oily Solution of Drug-Resistant Paediatric Epilepsies," paper presented to the Congress on Cannabis and the Cannabinoids, Leiden, The Netherlands, September 9–10, 2005; Resstel et al., "5-HT$_{1A}$ Receptors"; L. Weiss, M. Zeira, S. Reich, S. Slavin, I. Raz, R. Mechoulam, and R. Gallily, "Cannabidiol arrests onset of autoimmune diabetes in NOD mice," *Neuropharmacology* 54: 1 (January 2008), 244–49; Capasso et al., "Cannabidiol"; Malfait et al., "Nonpsychoactive Cannabis Constituent Cannabidiol"; Y. L. Hurd, M. Yoon, A. F. Manini, et al., "Early Phase in the Development of Cannabidiol as a Treatment for Addiction: Opioid Relapse Takes Initial Center Stage," *Neurotherapeutics* 12:4 (2015), 807–15; M. E. Sloan, J. L. Gowin, V. A. Ramchandani, Y. L. Hurd, and B. Le Foll, "The Endocannabinoid System as a Target for Addiction Treatment: Trials and Tribulations," *Neuropharmacology* 124 (September 15, 2017), 73–83, Reiman et al., "Cannabis as a Substitute"; J. R. Markos, H. M. Harris, W. Gul, M. A. ElSohly, and K. J. Sufka, "Effects of Cannabidiol on Morphine Conditioned Place Preference in Mice," *Planta Med.* August 9, 2017; Yasmin L. Hurd, "Cannabidiol: Swinging the Marijuana Pendulum From 'Weed' to Medication to Treat the Opioid Epidemic," *Trends Neurosci.* 40:3 (March 2017), 124–27.

293 Kentucky Department for Public Health, "Neonatal Abstinence Syndrome."

294 M. R. Grossman, A. K. Berkwitt, R. R. Osborn, Y. Xu, D. A. Esserman, E. D. Shapiro, and M. J. Bizzarro, "An Initiative to Improve the Quality of Care of Infants with Neonatal Abstinence Syndrome," *Pediatrics* pii:e20163360 (May 18, 2017), doi:10.1542/peds.2016-3360.

295 Caitlin Elizabeth Hughes and Alex Stevens, "What Can We Learn from the Portuguese Decriminalization of Illicit Drugs?" *British Journal of Criminology* 50:6 (November 1, 2010), 999–1022; Glenn Greenwald, "Drug Decriminalization in Portugal: Lessons for Creating Fair and Successful Drug Policies," white paper, Cato Institute, 2009.

296 Frederickson et al., "Correlation between the In Vivo and An In Vitro Expression."

297 Vela et al., "Anandamide Decreases Naloxone-Precipitated Withdrawal Signs."

298 Rubino et al., "Long-Term Treatment with SR141716A."

299 Mas-Nieto et al., "Reduction of Opioid Dependence."

300 SR141716A is an extremely potent CB1 receptor antagonist, with a K_i of 2.9 nM. McPartland et al., "Meta-analysis of Cannabinoid Ligand Binding Affinity."

301 Seely et al., "AM-251 and Rimonabant."

302 European Medicines Agency, "European Medicines Agency Recommends Suspension."

303 Moreira et al., "Psychiatric Side Effects"; European Medicines Agency, "Acomplia (Rimonabant)."

304 Yamaguchi et al., "Endogenous Cannabinoid, 2-Arachidonoylglycerol."

305 HU-210 is a potent CB1 agonist, with a mean K_i at human CB1 receptors of ~0.25 nM; McPartland et al., "Meta-analysis of Cannabinoid Ligand Binding Affinity."

306 Ibid.

307 Lichtman et al., "Opioid and Cannabinoid Modulation."

308 Valverde et al., "Delta-9-Tetrahydrocannabinol."

309 Del Arco et al., "Attenuation of Spontaneous Opiate Withdrawal."

310 Cichewicz et al., "Modulation of Oral Morphine Antinociceptive Tolerance."

311 Cox et al., "Synergy between Delta-9-Tetrahydrocannabinol and Morphine."

312 Abrams et al., "Cannabinoid-Opioid Interaction."

313 Collen et al., "Prescribing Cannabis"; Carter et al., "Cannabis in Palliative Medicine."

314 Scavone et al., "Cannabinoid and Opioid Interactions."

315 Bachhuber et al., "Medical Cannabis Laws."

316 Gruber et al., "Splendor in the Grass?"

317 Koob, "Dark Side of Emotion."

318 Crippa et al., "Therapeutical Use of the Cannabinoids."

319 Ibid.

320 Ibid.; Lewekel et al., "S39-02 Antipsychotic Effects of Cannabidiol."

321 Fernández-Ruiz et al., "Cannabidiol for Neurodegenerative Disorders."

322 Iuvone et al., "Cannabidiol"; Pelliccia et al., "Treatment with CBD."

323 Resstel et al., "5-HT1A Receptors."

324 Weiss et al., "Cannabidiol Arrests Onset."

325 Capasso et al., "Cannabidiol."

326 Malfait et al., "Nonpsychoactive Cannabis Constituent Cannabidiol."

327 Hurd et al., "Early Phase."

328 Sloan et al., "The Endocannabinoid System."

329 Reiman et al., "Cannabis as a Substitute."

330 Markos et al., "Effects of Cannabidiol."

331 Hurd, "Cannabidiol."

332 Kathmann et al., "Cannabidiol is an Allosteric Modulator."

333 Elizabeth S. Mezzacappa, E. S. Katkin, and S. N. Palmer, "Epinephrine, Arousal, and Emotion: A New Look at Two-Factor Theory," Cognition and Emotion 13:2 (1999), 181–99.

334 Arnau Busquets-Garcia, Maria Gomis-González, Raj Kamal Srivastava, Laura Cutando, Antonio Ortega-Alvaro, Sabine Ruehle, Floortje Remmers, et al., "Peripheral and Central CB1 Cannabinoid Receptors Control Stress-Induced Impairment of Memory Consolidation," PNAS 113:35 (2016), 9904–09; C. G. Ziegler, C. Mohn, V. Lamounier-Zepter, V.

Rettori, S. R. Bornstein, A. W. Krug, and M. Ehrhart-Bornstein, "Expression and Function of Endocannabinoid Receptors in the Human Adrenal Cortex," *Horm. Metab. Res.* 42:2 (Februar 2010), 88–92.

335 N. Niederhoffer, H. H. Hansen, J. J. Fernandez-Ruiz, and B. Szabo, "Effects of Cannabinoids on Adrenaline Release from Adrenal Medullary Cells," *British Journal of Pharmacology* 134:6 (2001), 1319–27; B. Malinowska, G. Godlewski, B. Bucher, E. Schlicker, "Cannabinoid CB1 Receptor-Mediated Inhibition of the Neurogenic Vasopressor Response in the Pithed Rat," *Naunyn-Schmiedeberg's Arch Pharmacol.* 356 (1997), 197–202; B. Szabo, U. Nordheim, and N. Niederhoffer, "Effects of Cannabinoids on Sympathetic and Parasympathetic Neuro-effector Transmission in the Rabbit Heart," *J. Pharmacol. Exp. Ther.* 297 (2001), 819–26.

336 P. Kienbaum, N. Thürauf, M. C. Michel, N. Scherbaum, M. Gastpar, and J. Peters, "Profound Increase in Epinephrine Concentration in Plasma and Cardiovascular Stimulation after Mu-Opioid Receptor Blockade in Opioid-Addicted Patients During Barbiturate-Induced Anesthesia for Acute Detoxification," *Anesthesiology* 88:5 (May 1998), 1154–61.

337 M. Hirokami, H. Togashi, M. Matsumoto, M. Yoshioka, and H. Saito, "The Functional Role of Opioid Receptors in Acetylcholine Release in the Rat Adrenal Medulla," *Eur. J. Pharmacol.* 253 (1994), 9–15; E. Gazyakan, M. Hennegriff, A. Haaf, G. B. Landwehrmeyer, T. J Feuerstein, and R. Jackisch, "Characterization of Opioid Receptor Types Modulating Acetylcholine Release in Septal Regions of the Rat Brain," *Naunyn-Schmiedeberg's Arch Pharmacol.* 362 (2000), 32–40; T. J. Feuerstein, O. Gleichauf, D. Peckys, G. B. Landwehrmeyer, R. Scheremet, and R. Jackisch, "Opioid Receptor-Mediated Control of Acetylcholine Release in Human Neocortex Tissue" *Naunyn-Schmiedeberg's Arch. Pharmacol.* 354 (2000), 586–92.

338 Del Arco et al., "Attenuation of Spontaneous Opiate Withdrawal"; Vela et al., "Anandamide Decreases Naloxone-Precipitated Withdrawal Signs"; Yamaguchi et al., "Endogenous Cannabinoid, 2-Arachidonoylglycerol."

339 J. Merrer, Jaj Becker, K. Befort, and B. Kieffer, "Reward Processing by the Opioid System in the Brain," *Physiological Reviews* 89:4 (2009), 1379–12.

340 A. Capasso, "GABA(B) Receptors Are Involved in the Control of Acute Opiate Withdrawal in Isolated Tissue," *Prog. Neuropsychopharmacol. Biol. Psychiatry* 23:2 (February 1999), 289–99; E. E. Bagley, M. B. Gerke, C. W. Vaughan, S. P. Hack, and M. J. Christie, "GABA Transporter Currents Activated by Protein Kinase A Excite Midbrain Neurons During Opioid Withdrawal," *Neuron* 45:3 (2005), 433–45.

341 Z. Sarnyai and G. L. Kovács, "Oxytocin in Learning and Addiction: From Early Discoveries to the Present," *Pharmacol. Biochem. Behav.* 119 (2014), 3–9; Z. Sarnyai and G. L. Kovács, "Role of Oxytocin in the Neuroadaptation to Drugs of Abuse," *Psychoneuroendocrinology* 19 (1994), 85–117.

342 U. Spampinato, E. Esposito, S. Romandini, et al., "Changes of Serotonin and Dopamine Metabolism in Various Forebrain Areas of Rats Injected with Morphine Either Systemically or in the Raphe Nuclei Dorsalis and Medianis," *Brain Res.* 328 (1985), 89–95; Bradley K. Taylor and Allan I. Basbaum, "Systemic Morphine-Induced Release of Serotonin in the Rostroventral Medulla is Not Mimicked by Morphine Microinjection into the Periaqueductal Gray," *Journal of Neurochemistry* 86 (2003), 1129–41; S. Kish, K. Kalasinsky, P. Derkach, et al., "Striatal Dopaminergic and Serotonergic Markers in Human Heroin Users," *Neuropsychopharmacology* 24 (2001), 561–67.

343 Monica Bawor, Herman Bami, Brittany B. Dennis, Carolyn Plater, Andrew Worster, Michael Varenbut, Jeff Daiter, et al., "Testosterone Suppression in Opioid Users: A Systematic Review and Meta-analysis," *Drug and Alcohol Dependence* 149 (April 1, 2015), 1–9.

344 M. R. Lashkarizadeh, M. Garshasbi, M. Shabani, S. Dabiri, H. Hadavi, and H. Manafi-Anari, "Impact of Opium Addiction on Levels of Pro- and Anti-inflammatory Cytokines after Surgery," *Addiction & Health* 8:1 (2016), 9–15; H. Yi, T. Iida, S. Liu, D. Ikegami, Q. Liu, A. Iida, D. A. Lubarsky, and S. Hao, "IL-4 Mediated by HSV Vector Suppresses Morphine Withdrawal Response and Decreases TNFα, NR2B, and pC/EBPβ in the Periaqueductal Gray in Rats," *Gene Therapy* 24 (April 2017), 224–33. P. Feng, J. J. Meissler Jr., M. W. Adler, and T. K. Eisenstein, "Morphine Withdrawal Sensitizes Mice to Lipopolysaccharide: Elevated TNF-alpha and Nitric Oxide with Decreased IL-12," *J. Neuroimmunol.* 164 (2005), 57–65; J. Kelschenbach, R. A. Barke, and S. Roy, "Morphine Withdrawal Contributes to Th2 Cell Differentiation by Biasing Cells Toward the Th2 Lineage," *J. Immunol.* 175 (2005), 2655–65.

345 Kalivas and Volkow, "Neural Basis of Addiction."

346 Kienbaum et al., "Profound Increase in Epinephrine Concentration."

347 B. Allolio, H. M. Schulte, U. Deuss, D. Kallabis, E. Hamel, W. Winkelman, "Effect of Oral Morphine and Naloxone on Pituitary-Adrenal Response in Man Induced by Human Corticotropin-Releasing Hormone," *Acta Endocrinologica* 114:4 (1987), 509–14.

348 J. Bearn, N. Buntwal, A. Papadopoulos, and S. Checkley, "Salivary Cortisol During Opiate Dependence and Withdrawal," *Addict. Biol.* 6:2 (April 2001), 157–62.

349 Nan-Jie Xu, Lan Bao, Hua-Ping Fan, Guo-Bin Bao, Lu Pu, Ying-Jin Lu, Chun-Fu Wu, et al., "Morphine Withdrawal Increases Glutamate Uptake and Surface Expression of Glutamate Transporter GLT1 at Hippocampal Synapses," *Journal of Neuroscience* 23:11 (June 1, 2003), 4775–84.

350 M. S. Gold, D. E. Redmond Jr., and H. D. Kleber, "Noradrenergic Hyperactivity in Opiate Withdrawal Supported by Clonidine Reversal of Opiate Withdrawal," *Am. J. Psychiatry* 136 (1979), 100–2; M. S. Gold, A. L. Pottash, and I. Extein, "Clonidine: Inpatient Studies from 1978 to 1981," *J. Clin. Psychiatry* 43 (1982), 35–8.

351 Hirokami et al., "Functional Role of Opioid Receptors"; Gazyakan et al., "Characterization of Opioid Receptor Types"; Feuerstein et al., "Opioid Receptor-Mediated Control."

352 H. L. Tripathi, F. J. Vocci, D. A. Brase, and W. L. Dewey, "Effects of Cannabinoids on Levels of Acetylcholine and Choline and on Turnover Rate of Acetylcholine in Various Regions of the Mouse Brain," *Alcohol Drug Res.* 7:5–6 (1987), 525–32; E. Acquas, A. Pisanu, P. Marrocu, and G. Di Chiara, "Cannabinoid CB1 Receptor Agonists Increase Rat Cortical and Hippocampal Acetylcholine Release In Vivo," *Eur. J. Pharmacol.* 401:2 (August 4, 2000), 179–85.

353 Viviana Trezza and Louk J. M. J. Vanderschuren, "Divergent Effects of Anandamide Transporter Inhibitors with Different Target Selectivity on Social Play Behavior in Adolescent Rats," *JPET* 328:1 (January 2009), 343–50.

354 E. Heyman, F. X. Gamelin, M. Goekint, F. Piscitelli, B. Roelands, E. Leclair, V. Di Marzo, and R. Meeusen, "Intense Exercise Increases Circulating Endocannabinoid and BDNF Levels in Humans—Possible Implications for Reward and Depression," *Psychoneuroendocrinology* 37:6 (June 2012), 844–51; D. A. Raichlen, A. D. Foster, G. L. Gerdeman, A. Seillier, and A. Giu Rida, "Wired to Run: Exercise-Induced Endocannabinoid Signaling in Humans and Cursorial Mammals with Implications for the 'Runner's High.'" *J. Exp. Biol.* 215 (April 15, 2012), 1331–36.

355 Del Arco et al., "Attenuation of Spontaneous Opiate Withdrawal"; Vela et al., "Anandamide Decreases Naloxone-Precipitated Withdrawal Signs"; Yamaguchi et al., "Endogenous Cannabinoid, 2-Arachidonoylglycerol."

356 R. J. Bluett, J. C. Gamble-George, D. J. Hermanson, N. D. Hartley, L. J. Marnett, and S. Patel, "Central Anandamide Deficiency Predicts Stress-Induced Anxiety: Behavioral Reversal through Endocannabinoid Augmentation, *Translational Psychiatry* 4:7 (2014). S. Kathuria, S. Gaetani, D. Fegley, F. Valino, A. Duranti, A. Tontini, et al., "Modulation of Anxiety through Blockade of Anandamide Hydrolysis," *Nat. Med.* 9 (2003), 76–81; O. Gunduz-Cinar, K. P. MacPherson, R. Cinar, J. Gamble-George, K. Sugden, B. Williams, et al., "Convergent Translational Evidence of a Role for Anandamide in Amygdala-Mediated Fear Extinction, Threat Processing and Stress-Reactivity," *Mol. Psychiatry* 18 (2013), 813–23.

357 S. J. Houser, M. Eads, J. P. Embrey, and S. P. Welch, "Dynorphin B and Spinal Analgesia: Induction of Antinociception by the Cannabinoids CP55,940, Delta(9)-THC and Anandamide," *Brain Res.* 857: 1–2 (February 28, 2000), 337–42.

358 Raichlen et al., "Wired to Run."

359 Houser et al., "Dynorphin B."

360 Kathmann et al., "Cannabidiol is an Allosteric Modulator."

361 Merrer et al., "Reward Processing."

362 Capasso, "GABA(B) Receptors"; Bagley et al., "GABA transporter Currents."

363 I. Ehrlich, Y. Humeau, F. Grenier, S. Ciocchi, C. Herry, and A. Lüthi, "Amygdala Inhibitory Circuits and the Control of Fear Memory," *Neuron* 62:6 (June 25, 2009), 757–71.

364 B. E. Alger, "Endocannabinoids and Their Implications for Epilepsy, *Epilepsy Currents* 4:5 (2004), 169–73.

365 C. C. Streeter, J. E. Jensen, R. M. Perlmutter, H. J. Cabral, H. Tian, D. B. Terhune, D. A. Ciraulo, and P. F. Renshaw, "Yoga Asana Sessions Increase Brain GABA Levels: A Pilot Study," *J. Altern. Complement. Med.* 13:4 (May 2007), 419–26.

366 L. E. Hill, S. K. Droste, D. J. Nutt, A. C. Linthorst, and J. M. Reul, "Voluntary Exercise Alters GABA(A) Receptor Subunit and Glutamic Acid Decarboxylase-67 Gene Expression in the Rat Forebrain," *J. Psychopharmacol.* 24:5 (May 2010), 745–56.

367 A. N. Elias, S. Guich, and A. F. Wilson, "Ketosis with Enhanced GABAergic Tone Promotes Physiological Changes in Transcendental Meditation," *Elsevier* 54:4 (April 2000), 660–62.

368 Sarnyai et al., "Oxytocin in learning"; Sarnyai et al., "Role of Oxytocin."

369 K. Nikolaou, D. Kapoukranidou, S. Ndungu, G. Floros, and L. Kovatsi, "Severity of Withdrawal Symptoms, Plasma Oxytocin Levels, and Treatment Outcome in Heroin Users Undergoing Acute Withdrawal," *J. Psychoactive Drugs* 49:3 (July–August 2017), 233–41.

370 G. L. Kovacs, Z. Sarnyai, and G. Szabo, "Oxytocin and Addiction: A Review," *Psychoneuroendocrinology* 23 (1998), 945–62.

371 I. D. Neumann, "The Advantage of Social Living: Brain Neuropeptides Mediate the Beneficial Consequences of Sex and Motherhood," *Front. Neuroendocrinol.* 30 (2009), 483–96; N. Magon and S. Kalra, "The Orgasmic History of Oxytocin: Love, Lust, and Labor," *Indian Journal of Endocrinology and Metabolism* 15:suppl. 3 (2011), S156–61.

372 M. S. Carmichael, V. L. Warburton, J. Dixen, and J. M. Davidson, "Relationship among Cardiovascular, Muscular, and Oxytocin Responses during Human Sexual Activity," *Arch. Sex. Behav.* 23 (1994), 59–79; M. S. Carmichael, R. Humbert, J. Dixen, G. Palmisano, W. Greenleaf, and J. M. Davidson, "Plasma Oxytocin Increases in the Human Sexual Response," *J. Clin. Endocrinol. Metab.* 64 (1987), 27–31.

373 K. M. Kendrick, "The Neurobiology of Social Bonds," *J. Neuroendocrinol.* 16 (2004), 1007–8.

374 Kosfeld et al., "Oxytocin Increases Trust."

375 Zak et al., "Oxytocin Increases Generosity."

376 Gunnar Rydén and Ingvar Sjöholm, "Half-Life of Oxytocin in Blood of Pregnant and Non-Pregnant Woman," *Acta Obstetricia et Gynecologica Scandinavica* 48: suppl. 3 (1969).

377 Don Wei, DaYeon Lee, Conor D. Cox, Carley A. Karsten, Olga Peñagarikano, Daniel H. Geschwind, Christine M. Gall, and Daniele Piomellia, "Endocannabinoid Signaling Mediates Oxytocin-Driven Social Reward," *PNAS* 112:45 (October 26, 2015), 14084–89.

378 Spampinato et al., "Changes of Serotonin"; Bradley et al., "Systemic Morphine-Induced Release."

379 Kish et al., "Striatal Dopaminergic and Serotonergic Markers."

380 E. Williams, B. Stewart-Knox, A. Helander, C. McConville, I. Bradbury, and I. Rowland, "Associations Between Whole-Blood Serotonin and Subjective Mood in Healthy

Male Volunteers," *Biol. Psychol.* 71:2 (February 2006), 171–74; A. R. Peirson and J. W. Heuchert, "Correlations for Serotonin Levels and Measures of Mood in a Nonclinical Sample," *Psychol. Rep.* 87:3 (December 2000), 707–16.

381 S. Haj-Dahmane and R. Y. Shen, "Modulation of the Serotonin System by Endocannabinoid Signaling," *Neuropharmacology* 61:3 (September 2011), 414–20.

382 Heyman et al., "Intense Exercise."

383 Allolio et al., "Effect of Oral Morphine."

384 Bearn et al., "Salivary Cortisol."

385 M. Walter, D. Bentz N. Schicktanz, A. Milnik, A. Aerni, C. Gerhards, K. Schwegler, et al., "Effects of Cortisol Administration on Craving in Heroin Addicts," *Translational Psychiatry* 5 (2015), e610.

386 S. Li, J. Li, D. H. Epstein, X. Y. Zhang, T. R. Kosten, and L. Lu, "Serum Cortisol Secretion During Heroin Abstinence Is Elevated Only Nocturnally," *American Journal of Drug and Alcohol Abuse* 34:3 (2008), 321–28.

387 T. L. Gruenewald, M. E. Kemeny, N. Aziz, and J. L. Fahey, "Acute Threat to the Social Self: Shame, Social Self-Esteem, and Cortisol Activity," *Psychosom. Med.* 66:6 (November–December 2004), 915–24.

388 J. Fernandez-Solari, J. P. Prestifilippo, P. Vissio, M. Ehrhart-Bornstein, S. R. Bornstein, V. Rettori, and J. C. Elverdin, "Anandamide Injected into the Lateral Ventricle of the Brain Inhibits Submandibular Salivary Secretion by Attenuating Parasympathetic Neurotransmission," *Braz. J. Med. Biol. Res.* 42:6 (June 2009), 537–44.

389 Gold et al., "Noradrenergic Hyperactivity"; Gold et al., "Clonidine: Inpatient Studies."

390 Kalivas et al., "Neural Basis of Addiction."

391 Bradley et al., "Systemic Morphine-Induced Release."

392 E. Gardner, "Endocannabinoid Signaling System and Brain Reward: Emphasis on Dopamine," *Pharmacol. Biochem. Behav.* 81 (2005), 263–84.

393 V. N. Salimpoor, M. Benovoy, K. Larcher, A. Dagher, and R. J. Zatorre, "Anatomically Distinct Dopamine Release during Anticipation and Experience of Peak Emotion to Music," *Nat. Neurosci.* 14:2 (February 2011), 257–62.

394 T. W. Kjaer, C. Bertelsen, P. Piccini, D. Brooks, J. Alving, and H. C. Lou, "Increased Dopamine Tone during Meditation-Induced Change of Consciousness," *Brain Res. Cogn. Brain Res.* 13:2 (April 2002), 255–59.

395 A. J. Hampson, M. Grimaldi, J. Axelrod, D. Wink, "Cannabidiol and (-)Δ9-Tetrahydrocannabinol are Neuroprotective Antioxidants," *Proceedings of the National Academy of Sciences of the USA* 95:14 (1998), 8268–73.

396 J. Mao, B. Sung, R. R. Ji, and G. Lim, "Chronic Morphine Induces Down Regulation of Spinal Glutamate Transporters: Implications in Morphine Tolerance and Abnormal Pain Sensitivity," *J. Neurosci.* 22 (2002), 8312–23.

397 Xu et al., "Morphine Withdrawal."

398 George K. Aghajanian, J. H. Kogan, and B. Moghaddam, "Opiate Withdrawal Increases Glutamate and Aspartate Efflux in the Locus Coeruleus: An In Vivo Microdialysis Study," *Brain Research* 636:1 (March 1994), 2630.

399 Ibid.

400 S. Aquila, C. Guido, A. Santoro, I. Perrotta, C. Laezza, M. Bifulco, et al., "Human Sperm Anatomy: Ultrastructural Localization of the Cannabinoid1 Receptor and a Potential Role of Anandamide in Sperm Survival and Acrosome Reaction," *Anat. Rec.* (Hoboken) 293:2 (2010), 298.

401 P. Grimaldi, D. Di Giacomo, R. Geremia, "The Endocannabinoid System and Spermatogenesis," *Frontiers in Endocrinology* 4 (2013), 192.

402 E. Agirregoitia, A. Carracedo, N. Subiran, A. Valdivia, N. Agirregoitia, L. Peralta, et al., "The CB(2) Cannabinoid Receptor Regulates Human Sperm Cell Motility," *Fertil. Steril.* 93:5 (2010), 1378–87; M. Rossato, F. Ion Popa, M. Ferigo, G. Clari, and C. Foresta, "Human Sperm Express Cannabinoid Receptor Cb1, the Activation of Which Inhibits Motility, Acrosome Reaction, and Mitochondrial Function," *J. Clin. Endocrinol. Metab.* 90:2 (2005), 984–91.

403 R. C. Kolodny, W. H. Masters, R. M. Kolodner, and G. Toro, "Depression of Plasma Testosterone Levels after Chronic Intensive Marihuana Use," *N. Engl. J. Med.* 290:16 (1974), 872–74.

404 G. Friedrich, W. Nepita, and T. Andre, "Serum Testosterone Concentrations in Cannabis and Opiate Users," *Beitr. Gerichtl. Med.* 48 (1990), 57–66; J. H. Mendelson, J. Kuehnle, J. Ellingboe, and T. F. Babor, "Plasma Testosterone Levels Before, During and After Chronic Marihuana Smoking," *N. Engl. J. Med.* 291:20 (1974), 1051–55; E. J. Cone, R. E Johnson, J. D. Moore, and J. D. Roache, "Acute Effects of Smoking Marijuana on Hormones, Subjective Effects and Performance in Male Human Subjects," *Pharmacol. Biochem. Behav.* 24:6 (1986), 1749–54.

405 N. Katz and N. A. Mazer, "The Impact of Opioids on the Endocrine System," *Clin. J. Pain* 25:2 (2009), 170–75.

406 Bawor et al., "Testosterone Suppression."

407 B. W. Craig, R. Brown, and J. Everhart, "Effects of Progressive Resistance Training on Growth Hormone and Testosterone Levels in Young and Elderly Subjects," *Mech. Ageing Dev.* 49:2 (August 1989), 159–69.

408 Nandini Acharya, Sasi Penukonda, Tatiana Shcheglova, Adam T. Hagymasi, Sreyashi Basu, and Pramod K. Srivastava, "Endocannabinoid System Acts as a Regulator of Immune Homeostasis in the Gut," *PNAS* 114:19 (2017), 5005–10; R. Pandey, K. Mousawy, M. Nagarkatti, and P. Nagarkatti, "Endocannabinoids and Immune Regulation," *Pharmacological Research* 60:2 (2009), 85–92.

409 Lashkarizadeh et al., "Impact of Opium Addiction."

410 Yi et al., "IL-4 Mediated by HSV Vector.""

411 Feng et al., "Morphine Withdrawal"; Kelschenbach et al., "Morphine Withdrawal."

412 Chi-Mei Ku and Jin-Yuarn Lin, "Anti-inflammatory Effects of 27 Selected Terpenoid Compounds Tested Through Modulating Th1/Th2 Cytokine Secretion Profiles Using Murine Primary Splenocytes," *Food Chemistry* 141:2 (November 15, 2013), 1104–13.

413 J. D. Creswell, M. R. Irwin, L. J. Burklund, et al., "Mindfulness-Based Stress Reduction Training Reduces Loneliness and Pro-Inflammatory Gene Expression in Older Adults: A Small Randomized Controlled Trial," *Brain, Behavior, and Immunity* 26:7 (2012), 1095–110.

414 M. Lijffijt, K. Hu, and A. C. Swann, "Stress Modulates Illness-Course of Substance Use Disorders: A Translational Review," *Frontiers in Psychiatry* 5 (2014), 83.

415 A. Armario, "Activation of the Hypothalamic-Pituitary-Adrenal Axis by Addictive Drugs: Different Pathways, Common Outcome," *Trends Pharmacol. Sci.* 31:7 (July 2010), 318–25.

416 G. Wand, "The Influence of Stress on the Transition From Drug Use to Addiction," *Alcohol Research & Health* 31:2 (2008), 119–36.

417 Kathryn Hausknecht, Samir Haj-Dahmane, and Roh-Yu Shen, "Prenatal Stress Exposure Increases the Excitation of Dopamine Neurons in the Ventral Tegmental Area and Alters Their Reponses to Psychostimulants," *Neuropsychopharmacology* 38 (2013), 293–301.

418 E. Charmandari, T. Kino, E. Souvatzoglou, G. P. Chrousos, "Pediatric Stress: Hormonal Mediators and Human Development," *Horm. Res.* 59 (2003), 161–79.

419 K. Mizoguchi, A. Ishige, M. Aburada, and T. Tabira, "Chronic Stress Attenuates Glucocorticoid Negative Feedback: Involvement of the Prefrontal Cortex and Hippocampus," *Neuroscience* 119:3 (2003), 887–97.

420 Charmandari et al., "Pediatric Stress."

421 Stanislav Grof, *Beyond the Brain: Birth, Death, and Transendence in Psychotherapy* (Albany, NY: State University of New York Press, 1985); Stanislav Grof, *Healing Our Deepest Wounds: The Holotropic Paradigm Shift* (Newcastle, WA: Stream of Experience, 2012).

422 Frédérick Leboyer, *Birth without Violence,* 4th ed. (New York: Healing Arts Press, 2009).

423 Lloyd DeMause, *Emotional Life of Nations* (New York: Karnac, 2002), http://psychohistory .com/books/the-emotional-life-of-nations.

424 Minton et al., "Drug Related Deaths in Scotland."

425 U.S. CDC, "Today's Heroin Epidemic Infographics," Vital Signs, http://www.cdc.gov /vitalsigns/heroin/infographic.html.

426 Minton et al., "Drug Related Deaths in Scotland."

427 "Apartheid, Perpetrators, Forgiveness: Desmond Tutu's Views," http://www.youtube.com /watch?v=eRDBWoV_hA0.

428 Giacomo Bono and Michael E. McCullough, "Positive Responses to Benefit and Harm: Bringing Forgiveness and Gratitude Into Cognitive Psychotherapy," *Journal of Cognitive Psychotherapy* 20:2 (2006); C. V. Witvliet, T. E. Ludwig, and D. J. Bauer, "Please Forgive Me: Transgressors' Emotions and Physiology during Imagery of Seeking Forgiveness and Victim Responses," *Journal of Psychology and Christianity* 21 (2002), 219–33.

429 Sidney Piburn, *The Dalai Lama, a Policy of Kindness: An Anthology of Writings by and About the Dalai Lama* (Delhi: Motilal Banarsidass, 1997), 99.

430 Hughes et al., "Resounding Success."

431 Bachhuber, "Medical Cannabis Laws."

432 European Monitoring Centre for Drugs and Drug Addiction, "Portugal: Country Drug Report," 2017, doi:10.2810/457245.

433 Flor et al., "Efficacy of Multidisciplinary Pain Treatment Centers"; Roberts et al., "Behavioral Management"; Kamper et al., "Multidisciplinary Biopsychosocial Rehabilitation"; Patrick et al., "Long-Term Outcomes"; J. J. Chen, "Outpatient Pain Rehabilitation Programs," *Iowa Orthopaedic Journal* 26 (2006), 102–6.

434 B. K. Alexander, "The Globalization of Addiction," *Addiction Research* 8 (2000), 501–26.

435 B. K. Alexander, R. B. Coambs, and P. F. Hadaway, "The Effect of Housing and Gender on Morphine Self-Administration in Rats," *Psychopharmacology* 58 (1978), 175–79.

436 Alexander, "Globalization of Addiction."

437 L. R. Stanley, S. D. Harness, R. C. Swaim, F. Beauvais, "Rates of Substance Use of American Indian Students in 8th, 10th, and 12th Grades Living on or Near Reservations: Update, 2009–2012," *Public Health Reports* 129:2 (2014), 156–63.

438 Johann Hari, *Chasing the Scream: The First and Last Days on the War on Drugs* (New York: Bloomsbury, 2015).

439 Johann Hari, "Everything You Think You Know about Addiction Is Wrong," TED Talk, June 2015, http://goo.gl/kbcBSX.

440 S. Bowen, N. Chawla, S. E. Collins, et al., "Mindfulness-Based Relapse Prevention for Substance Use Disorders: A Pilot Efficacy Trial," *Substance Abuse* 30:4 (2009), 295–305.

441 J. L. Riley, B. A. Hastie, T. L. Glover, C. M. Campbell, R. Staud, R. B. Fillingim, "Cognitive-Affective and Somatic Side Effects of Morphine and Pentazocine: Side-Effect Profiles in Healthy Adults," *Pain Medicine* 11:2 (2010), 10.

442 R. E. Balter and M. Haney, chap. 85, "The Synthetic Analog of Δ9-Tetrahydrocannabinol (THC): Nabilone. Pharmacology and Clinical Application," *Handbook of Cannabis and Related Pathologies: Biology, Pharmacology, Diagnosis, and Treatment* (New York: Elsevier, 2017), 821–27.

443 Method acting emerged out of the teachings of the Russian theater director Konstantin Sergeievich Stanislavski, in which actors are taught techniques such as learning to match a mental-emotional expression while playing a part with that of an actual experience. Another technique would be to learn everything one could about a person who had the experience, including their culture, psychology (beliefs, attitudes, thoughts, feeling, decisions, choices), and resulting behavior and to act "as if." The latter technique includes exercises such as developing "as if" sensory memory in great detail, and in essence becoming or at least approximating becoming that person in the way they think, feel, and act.

444 Beal et al., "Dronabinol as a Treatment for Anorexia."

445 Multidisciplinary Association for Psychedelic Studies, "FDA Grants Breakthrough Therapy Designation for MDMA-Assisted Psychotherapy for PTSD, Agrees on Special Protocol Assessment for Phase 3 Trials," press release, August 26, 2017, http://goo.gl/VNrCi1; M. C. Mithoefer, M. T.Wagner, A. T. Mithoefer, L. Jerome, and R. J. Doblin, "Durability of Improvement in Post–Traumatic Stress Disorder Symptoms and Absence of Harmful Effects or Drug Dependency after 3,4-Methylenedioxymethamphetamine-Assisted Psychotherapy: A Prospective Long-Term Follow-up Study," *Psychopharmacol.* 25 (2011), 439–52.

446 Roland R. Griffiths, Matthew W. Johnson, Michael A. Carducci, Annie Umbricht, William A. Richards, Brian D. Richards, Mary P. Cosimano, and Margaret A. Klinedinst, "Psilocybin Produces Substantial and Sustained Decreases in Depression and Anxiety in Patients with Life-Threatening Cancer: A Randomized Double-Blind Trial, *Journal of Psychopharmacology* 30:12 (2016); C. S. Grob, A. L. Danforth, and G. S. Chopra, "Pilot Study of Psilocybin Treatment for Anxiety in Patients with Advanced-Stage Cancer, *Arch. Gen. Psychiatry* 68 (2011), 71–78.

447 P. Gasser, D. Holstein, and Y. Michel, "Safety and Efficacy of Lysergic Acid Diethylamide-Assisted Psychotherapy for Anxiety Associated with Life-Threatening Diseases," *Journal Nerv. Ment. Dis.* 202 (2014), 513–20.

448 T. K. Brown, "Ibogaine in the Treatment of Substance Dependence," *Curr. Drug Abuse Rev.* 6:1 (March 2013), 3–16; S. D. Glick and I. S. Maisonneuve, "Mechanisms of Antiaddictive Actions of Ibogaine," *Ann. NY Acad. Sci.*844 (1998), 214–26; T. Antonio, S. R. Childers, R. B. Rothman, C. M. Dersch, C. King, M. Kuehne, W. G. Bornmann, et al., "Effect of Iboga Alkaloids on Micro-opioid Receptor-Coupled G Protein Activation," *PLoS One* 2013, 8:e77262.

449 S. Wright, P. Duncombe, D. G. Altman, "Assessment of Blinding to Treatment Allocation in Studies of a Cannabis-Based Medicine (Sativex) in People with Multiple Sclerosis: A New Approach," *Trials* 13 (2012), 189.

450 B. K. O'Connell, D. Gloss, and O. Devinsky, "Cannabinoids in Treatment-Resistant Epilepsy: A Review," *Epilepsy Behav.* 70:pt. B (May 2017), 341–48.

451 Bergamaschi et al., "Safety and Side Effects of Cannabidiol."

BIBLIOGRAPHY

Abdel-Salam, Omar. "Gastric Acid Inhibitory and Gastric Protective Effects of Cannabis and Cannabinoids," *Asian Pacific Journal of Tropical Medicine* 9:5 (May 2016), 413–19.

Abrams, D. I., C. A. Jay, S. B. Shade, H. Vizoso, H. Reda, S. Press, M. E. Kelly, et al. "Cannabis in Painful HIV-Associated Sensory Neuropathy: A Randomized Placebo-Controlled Trial," *Neurology* 68:7 (February 13, 2007), 515–21.

Abrams, D. I., P. Couey, S. B. Shade, M. E. Kelly, N. L. Benowitz. "Cannabinoid-Opioid Interaction in Chronic Pain," *Clin. Pharmacol. Ther.* 90:6 (December 2011), 844–51.

Abs, R., J. Verhelst, J. Maeyaert, J. P. Van Buyten, F. Opsomer, H. Adriaensen, Jan Verlooy, Tony Van Havenbergh, Mike Smet, and Kristien Van Acker. "Endocrine Consequences of Long-Term Intrathecal Administration of Opioids," *J. Clin. Endocrinol. Metab.* 85 (2000), 2215–22.

Acharya, Nandini, Sasi Penukonda, Tatiana Shcheglova, Adam T. Hagymasi, Sreyashi Basu, and Pramod K. Srivastava. "Endocannabinoid System Acts as a Regulator of Immune Homeostasis in the Gut," *PNAS* 114:19 (2017), 5005–10.

Acquas, E., A. Pisanu, P. Marrocu, and G. Di Chiara. "Cannabinoid CB1 Receptor Agonists Increase Rat Cortical and Hippocampal Acetylcholine Release In Vivo," *Eur. J. Pharmacol.* 401:2 (August 4, 2000), 179–85.

Adams, P. M., and E. S. Barratt. "Effect of Chronic Marijuana Administration of Stages of Primate Sleep-Wakefulness," *Biol. Psychiatry* 10:3 (June 1975), 315–22.

Agarwal, N., P. Pacher, I. Tegeder, et al. "Cannabinoids Mediate Analgesia Largely Via Peripheral Type 1 Cannabinoid Receptors in Nociceptors, *Nature Neuroscience*10:7 (2007), 870–79.

Agarwal, N., P. Pacher, I. Tegeder, F. Amaya, C. E. Constantin, G. J. Brenner, T. Rubino, et al. "Cannabinoids Mediate Analgesia Largely Via Peripheral Type 1 Cannabinoid Receptors in Nociceptors," *Nat. Neurosci.* 10 (2007), 870–79.

Aghajanian, George K., J. H. Kogan, and B. Moghaddam. "Opiate Withdrawal Increases Glutamate and Aspartate Efflux in the Locus Coeruleus: An In Vivo Microdialysis Study," *Brain Research* 636:1 (March 1994), 2630.

Agirregoitia, E., A. Carracedo, N. Subiran, A. Valdivia, N. Agirregoitia, L. Peralta, et al. "The CB(2) Cannabinoid Receptor Regulates Human Sperm Cell Motility," *Fertil. Steril.* 93:5 (2010), 1378–87.

Akopian, A. N., N. B. Ruparel, N. A. Jeske, A. Patwardhan, and K. M. Hargreaves. "Role of Ionotropic Cannabinoid Receptors in Peripheral Antinociception and Antihyperalgesia," *Trends Pharmacol. Sci.* 30 (2009), 79–84.

Alexander, B. K. "The Globalization of Addiction," *Addiction Research* 8 (2000), 501–26.

Alexander, B. K., R. B. Coambs, and P. F. Hadaway. "The Effect of Housing and Gender on Morphine Self-Administration in Rats," *Psychopharmacology* 58 (1978), 175–79.

Alger, B. E. "Endocannabinoids and Their Implications for Epilepsy, *Epilepsy Currents* 4:5 (2004), 169–73.

Algren, D., C. Monteilh, C. Rubin, et al. "Fentanyl-Associated Fatalities among Illicit Drug Users in Wayne County, Michigan (July 2005–May 2006)," *Journal of Medical Toxicology* 9:1 (March 2013), 106–15.

Allolio, B., H. M. Schulte, U. Deuss, D. Kallabis, E. Hamel, W. Winkelman. "Effect of Oral Morphine and Naloxone on Pituitary-Adrenal Response in Man Induced by Human Corticotropin-Releasing Hormone," *Acta Endocrinologica* 114:4 (1987), 509–14.

American Civil Liberties Union. "Finding 4: Blacks and Whites Use Marijuana at Similar Rates," *The War on Marijuana in Black and White*, June 2013, 21.

American Psychiatric Association. *Diagnostic and Statistical Manual of Mental Disorders,* 5th ed. (*DSM-5*). Arlington, VA: American Psychiatric Publishing, 2013.

Anslinger, H. J., and W. F. Tompkins. *The Traffic in Narcotics.* New York: Funk and Wagnalls, 1953.

Anthony, James C., Lynn A. Warner, and Ronald C. Kessler. "Comparative Epidemiology of Dependence on Tobacco, Alcohol, Controlled Substances, and Inhalants: Basic Findings from the National Comorbidity Survey," *Experimental and Clinical Psychopharmacology* 2:3 (1994), 244–68.

Antonio, T., S. R. Childers, R. B. Rothman, C. M. Dersch, C. King, M. Kuehne, W. G. Bornmann, et al. "Effect of Iboga Alkaloids on Micro-opioid Receptor-Coupled G Protein Activation," *PLoS One* 2013, 8:e77262.

Aquila, S., C. Guido, A. Santoro, I. Perrotta, C. Laezza, M. Bifulco, et al. "Human Sperm Anatomy: Ultrastructural Localization of the Cannabinoid1 Receptor and a Potential Role of Anandamide in Sperm Survival and Acrosome Reaction," *Anat. Rec.* (Hoboken) 293:2 (2010), 298.

Aristotle. Historia Animalium.

———. Physica Minora.

Armario, A. "Activation of the Hypothalamic-Pituitary-Adrenal Axis by Addictive Drugs: Different Pathways, Common Outcome," *Trends Pharmacol. Sci.* 31:7 (July 2010), 318–25.

Arnér, S., and B. A. Meyerson. "Lack of Analgesic Effect Of opioids on Neuropathic and Idiopathic Forms of Pain," *Pain* 33:1 (April 1988), 11–23.

Ashton, C. H., P. B. Moore, P. Gallagher, and A. H. Young. "Cannabinoids in Bipolar Affective Disorder: A Review and Discussion of Their Therapeutic Potential," *J. Psychopharmacol.* 19:3 (May 2005), 293–300.

Ashton, J. C., and M. Glass. "The Cannabinoid CB2 Receptor as a Target for Inflammation-Dependent Neurodegeneration," *Current Neuropharmacology* 5:2 (2007), 73–80.

Ashton, J. C., and P. F. Smith. "Cannabinoids and Cardiovascular Disease: The Outlook for Clinical Treatments," *Curr. Vasc. Pharmacol.* 5:3 (July 2007), 175–85.

Askitopoulou, Helen, Ioanna A. Ramoutsaki, and Eleni Konsolaki. "Analgesia and Anesthesia: The Etymology and Literary History of Related Greek Words," *Analgesia & Anesthesia* 91:2 (2000), 486–91.

———. "Archaeological Evidence on the Use of Opium in the Minoan World," *International Congress Series* 1242 (December 2002), 23–29.

Askwith, R. "How Aspirin Turned Hero," *Sunday Times* (London), September 13, 1998.

Attal, N., L. Brasseur, D. Guirimand, S. Clermond-Gnamien, S. Atlami, and D. Bouhassira. "Are Oral Cannabinoids Safe and Effective in Refractory Neuropathic Pain?" *Eur. J. Pain* 8:2 (April 2004), 173–77.

Bachhuber, M. A., B. Saloner, C. O. Cunningham, and C. L. Barry. "Medical Cannabis Laws and Opioid Analgesic Overdose Mortality in the United States, 1999–2010," *JAMA Internal Medicine* 174:10 (2014), 1668–73.

Bagley, E. E., M. B. Gerke, C. W. Vaughan, S. P. Hack, and M. J. Christie. "GABA Transporter Currents Activated by Protein Kinase A Excite Midbrain Neurons During Opioid Withdrawal," *Neuron* 45:3 (2005), 433–45.

Bahi, A., S. Mansouri, E. Memari, M. Ameri, S. M. Nurulain, and S. Ojha. "⊠-Caryophyllene, a CB2 Receptor Agonist Produces Multiple Behavioral Changes Relevant to Anxiety and Depression in Mice," *Physiol. Behav.* 135 (August 2014), 119–24.

Ballantyne, J. C. "Opioid Analgesia: Perspectives on Right Use and Utility," *Pain Physician* 10 (2007), 479–91.

Ballantyne, J. C., and J. Mao. "Opioid Therapy for Chronic Pain," *N. Engl. J. Med.* 349 (2003), 1943–53.

Balter, R. E., and M. Haney. "The Synthetic Analog of Δ9-Tetrahydrocannabinol (THC): Nabilone. Pharmacology and Clinical Application," *Handbook of Cannabis and Related Pathologies: Biology, Pharmacology, Diagnosis, and Treatment.* New York: Elsevier, 2017, 821–27.

Bambico, F. R., N. Katz, G. Debonnel, and G. Gobbi. "Cannabinoids Elicit Antidepressant-like Behavior and Activate Serotonergic Neurons through the Medial Prefrontal Cortex," *J. Neurosci.* 27:43 (2007), 11700–11.

Bambico, F. R., P. R. Hattan, J. P. Garant, and G. Gobbi. "Effect of Delta-9-Tetrahydrocannabinol on Behavioral Despair and on Pre- and Postsynaptic Serotonergic Transmission," *Prog. Neuropsychopharmacol. Biol. Psychiatry* 38:1 (July 2, 2012), 88–96.

Baum, Dan. "Legalize It All: How to Win the War on Drugs," *Harper's Magazine*, April 2016.

Bawor, Monica, Herman Bami, Brittany B. Dennis, Carolyn Plater, Andrew Worster, Michael Varenbut, Jeff Daiter, et al. "Testosterone Suppression in Opioid Users: A Systematic Review and Meta-analysis," *Drug and Alcohol Dependence* 149 (April 1, 2015), 1–9.

Bayer and GW Pharmaceutical. "Sativex Oromucosal Spray." Patient information leaflet. May 20, 2015.

Beal, J. E., R. Olson, L. Laubenstein, J. O. Morales, P. Bellman, B. Yangco, L. Lefkowitz, et al. "Dronabinol as a Treatment for Anorexia Associated with Weight Loss in Patients with AIDS," *Journal of Pain and Symptom Management* 10:2 (1995), 89–97.

Bearn, J., N. Buntwal, A. Papadopoulos, and S. Checkley. "Salivary Cortisol During Opiate Dependence and Withdrawal," *Addict. Biol.* 6:2 (April 2001), 157–62.

Beauchamp, G. A., E. L. Winstanley, S. A. Ryan, and M. S. Lyons. "Moving Beyond Misuse and Diversion: The Urgent Need to Consider the Role of Iatrogenic Addiction in the Current Opioid Epidemic," *American Journal of Public Health* 104:11 (2014), 2023–29.

Beaumont, H., J. Jensen, A. Carlsson, M. Ruth, A. Lehmann, and G. E. Boeckx-staens. "Effect of Delta(9)-Tetrahydrocannabinol, a Cannabinoid Receptor Agonist, on the Triggering of Transient Lower Esoesophageal Sphincter Relaxations in Dogs and Humans," *Br. J. Pharmacol.* 156:1 (January 2009), 153–62.

Beecher, H. K. "Relationship of Significance of Wound to Pain Experienced," *JAMA* 161:17 (August 1956), 1609–13.

Bento, A. F., R. Marcon, R. C. Dutra, et al. "☐-Caryophyllene Inhibits Dextran Sulfate Sodium-Induced Colitis in Mice through CB2 Receptor Activation and PPAR☐ Pathway," *American Journal of Pathology* 178:3 (2011), 1153–66.

Bergamaschi, Mateus Machado, Regina Helena Costa Queiroz, José Alexandre S. Crippa, and Antonio Waldo Zuardi. "Safety and Side Effects of Cannabidiol, a Cannabis sativa Constituent," *Current Drug Safety* 6:4 (2011).

Bergmann, Karl-Christian. "Dronabinol—eine mögliche neue erapie- option bei COPD-Patienten mit pulmonaler Kachexie," paper presented at the 2005 Conference of the German Society for Pneumology, Berlin, March 17, 2005.

Berman, J. S., C. Symonds, and R. Birch. "Efficacy of Two Cannabis-Based Medicinal Extracts for Relief of Central Neuropathic Pain from Brachial Plexus Avulsion: Results of a Randomised Controlled Trial," *Pain* 112:3 (2004), 299–306.

Bisaga, A., M. A. Sullivan, A. Glass, et al. "The Effects of Dronabinol During Detoxification and the Initiation of Treatment With Extended Release Naltrexone," *Drug and Alcohol Dependence* 154 (2015), 38–45.

Bisogno, T., L. Hanus, L. De Petrocellis, S. Tchilibon, D. E. Ponde, I. Brandi, et al. "Molecular Targets for Cannabidiol and Its Synthetic Analogues: Effect on Vanilloid VR1 Receptors and on the Cellular Uptake and Enzymatic Hydrolysis of Anandamide," *Br. J. Pharmacol.* 134 (2001), 845–52.

Blake, D. R., P. Robson, M. Ho, R. W. Jubb, and C. S. McCabe. "Preliminary Assessment of the Efficacy, Tolerability and Safety of a Cannabis-Based Medicine (Sativex) in the Treatment of Pain Caused by Rheumatoid Arthritis," *Rheumatology* 45:1 (2006), 50–52.

Bluett, R. J., J. C. Gamble-George, D. J. Hermanson, N. D. Hartley, L. J. Marnett, and S. Patel. "Central Anandamide Deficiency Predicts Stress-Induced Anxiety: Behavioral Reversal through Endocannabinoid Augmentation, *Translational Psychiatry* 4:7 (2014).

Bluett, Rebecca J., Rita Báldi, Andre Haymer, Andrew D. Gaulden, Nolan D. Hartley, Walker P. Parrish, Jordan Baechle, et al. "Endocannabinoid Signalling Modulates Susceptibility to Traumatic Stress Exposure," *Nature Communications* 8, article no. 14782 (2017).

Boecker, H, T. Sprenger, M. E. Spilker, G. Henriksen, M. Koppenhoefer, K. J. Wagner, M. Valet, A. Berthele, and T. R. Tolle, "The Runner's High: Opioidergic Mechanisms in the Human Brain," *Cerebral Cortex* 18:11 (November 2008), 2523–31.

Bono, Giacomo, and Michael E. McCullough. "Positive Responses to Benefit and Harm: Bringing Forgiveness and Gratitude Into Cognitive Psychotherapy," *Journal of Cognitive Psychotherapy* 20:2 (2006).

Boorman, Emily, Zuzanna Zajkowska, Rumsha Ahmed, Carmine M. Pariante, and Patricia A. Zunszain. "Crosstalk between Endocannabinoid and Immune Systems: A Potential Dysregulation in Depression?" *Psychopharmacology* (Berl). 233 (2016), 1591–1604.

Booz, George W. "Cannabidiol as an Emergent Therapeutic Strategy for Lessening the Impact of Inflammation on Oxidative Stress," *Free Radic. Biol. Med.* 51:5 (September 1, 2011), 1054–61.

Borrelli, F., G. Aviello, B. Romano, P. Orlando, R. Capasso, F. Maiello, F. Guadagno, et al. "Cannabidiol, a Safe and NonPsychotropic Ingredient of the Marijuana Plant *Cannabis sativa,* Is Protective in a Murine Model Of Colitis," *J. Mol. Med.* (Berl). 87:11 (November 2009), 1111–21.

Bowen, S., N. Chawla, S. E. Collins, et al. "Mindfulness-Based Relapse Prevention for Substance Use Disorders: A Pilot Efficacy Trial," *Substance Abuse* 30:4 (2009), 295–305.

Brady, K. T., P. Tuerk, S. E. Back, M. E. Saladin, A. E. Waldrop, H. Myrick. "Combat Posttraumatic Stress Disorder, Substance Use Disorders, and Traumatic Brain Injury," *Journal of Addiction Medicine* 3:4 (2009), 179–88.

Bremner, J. D., S. M Southwick, A. Darnell, and D. S. Charney. "Chronic PTSD in Vietnam Combat Veterans: Course of Illness and Substance Abuse," *Am. J. Psychiatry* 153:3 (March 1996), 369–75.

Brierley, D. I., J. Samuels, M. Duncan, B. J. Whalley, and C. M. Williams. "Cannabigerol Is a Novel, Well-Tolerated Appetite Stimulant in Pre-satiated Rats," *Psychopharmacology* 2016;233(19):3603-3613.

———. "A Cannabigerol-Rich Cannabis Sativa Extract, Devoid of 9-Tetrahydrocannabinol, Elicits Hyperphagia in Rats," *Behav. Pharmacol.* 28:4 (June 2017), 280–84.

Britch, S. C., J. L. Wiley, Z. Yu, B. H. Clowers, and R. M. Craft. "Cannabidiol-Δ9-Tetrahydrocannabinol Interactions on Acute Pain and Locomotor Activity," *Drug Alcohol Depend.* 175 (June 1, 2017), 187–97.

Brown, T. K. "Ibogaine in the Treatment of Substance Dependence," *Curr. Drug Abuse Rev.* 6:1 (March 2013), 3–16.

Brown, Thomas. "The Hypodermic or Subcutaneous Syringe," in *Alexander Wood: A sketch of His Life and Work*. Edinburgh: Macniven & Wallace, 1886, 107–114.

Brusberg, M., S. Arvidsson, D. Kang, H. Larsson, E. Lindström, and V. Martinez. "CB1 Receptors Mediate the Analgesic Effects of Cannabinoids on Colorectal Distension-Induced Visceral Pain in Rodents," *J. Neurosci.* 29:5 (February 4, 2009), 1554–64.

Burstein, Sumner H., and Robert B. Zurier. "Cannabinoids, Endocannabinoids, and Related Analogs in Inflammation," *AAPS J.* 11:1 (March 2009), 109–19.

Burstein, Sumner. "Ajulemic Acid (IP-751): Synthesis, Proof of Principle, Toxicity Studies, and Clinical Trials," *AAPS J.* 7:1 (March 2005), E143–48.

Busquets-Garcia, Arnau, Maria Gomis-González, Raj Kamal Srivastava, Laura Cutando, Antonio Ortega-Alvaro, Sabine Ruehle, Floortje Remmers, et al. "Peripheral and Central CB1 Cannabinoid Receptors Control Stress-Induced Impairment of Memory Consolidation," *PNAS* 113:35 (2016), 9904–09.

Campbell, J. N. "APS 1995 Presidential address," *Pain Forum* 5 (1996) 85–8.

Campos, A. C., M. V. Fogaça, A. B. Sonego, and F. S. Guimarães. "Cannabidiol, Neuroprotection and Neuropsychiatric Disorders," *Pharmacol. Res.* 112 (October 2016), 119–27.

Campos, Alline C., Manoela V. Fogaça, Franciele F. Scarante, Sâmia R. L. Joca, Amanda J. Sales, Felipe V. Gomes, Andreza B. Sonego, et al. "Plastic and Neuroprotective Mechanisms Involved in the Therapeutic Effects of Cannabidiol in Psychiatric Disorders," *Front. Pharmacol.* May 23, 2017.

Campos, Alline Cristina, Fabricio Araújo Moreira, Felipe Villela Gomes, Elaine Aparecida Del Bel, and Francisco Silveira Guimarães. "Multiple Mechanisms Involved in the Large-Spectrum Therapeutic Potential of Cannabidiol in Psychiatric Disorders," *Philos. Trans. R. Soc. Lond. B Biol. Sci.* 367:1607 (December 5, 2012).

Capasso, A. "GABA(B) Receptors Are Involved in the Control of Acute Opiate Withdrawal in Isolated Tissue," *Prog. Neuropsychopharmacol. Biol. Psychiatry* 23:2 (February 1999), 289–99.

Capasso, R., F. Borrelli, G. Aviello, B. Romano, C. Scalisi, F. Capasso, and A. Izzo. "Cannabidiol, Extracted from *Cannabis sativa*, Selectively Inhibits in Ammatory Hypermotility in Mice," *Br. J. Pharmacol.* 154:5 (July 2008), 1001–08.

Carlini, E. A., and J. M. Cunha. "Hypnotic and Antiepileptic Effects of Cannabidiol," *J. Clin. Pharmacol.* 21:8–9 suppl. (August–September 1981), 417S–427S.

Carmichael, M. S., R. Humbert, J. Dixen, G. Palmisano, W. Greenleaf, and J. M. Davidson. "Plasma Oxytocin Increases in the Human Sexual Response," *J. Clin. Endocrinol. Metab.* 64 (1987), 27–31.

Carmichael, M. S., V. L. Warburton, J. Dixen, and J. M. Davidson. "Relationship among Cardiovascular, Muscular, and Oxytocin Responses during Human Sexual Activity," *Arch. Sex. Behav.* 23 (1994), 59–79.

Carter, G. T., A. M. Flanagan, M. Earleywine, D. I. Abrams, S. K. Aggarwal, and L. Grinspoon. "Cannabis in Palliative Medicine: Improving Care and Reducing Opioid-Related Morbidity," *Am. J. Hosp. Palliat. Care* 28 (2011), 297–303.

Carter, Gregory T., Patrick Weydt, Muraco Kyashna-Tocha, and Donald Abrams. "Medicinal Cannabis: Rational Guidelines for Dosing," *IDrugs* 7:5 (May 2004), 464–70.

Center for Behavioral Health Statistics and Quality. *2014 National Survey on Drug Use and Health: Detailed Tables* Rockville, MD: Substance Abuse and Mental Health Services Administration, 2015.

———. *Key Substance Use and Mental Health Indicators in the United States: Results from the 2015 National Survey on Drug Use and Health,* HHS Publication SMA 16-4984 (2016), 21.

Charmandari, E., T. Kino, E. Souvatzoglou, G. P. Chrousos. "Pediatric Stress: Hormonal Mediators and Human Development," *Horm. Res.* 59 (2003), 161–79.

Chemical Heritage Foundation. "Felix Hoffmann," www.chemheritage.org/historical-profile /felix-hoffmann. Accessed September 10, 2017.

Chen, J. J. "Outpatient Pain Rehabilitation Programs," *Iowa Orthopaedic Journal* 26 (2006), 102–6.

Chen, L., J. Zhang, F. Li, Y. Qiu, L. Wang, Y. H. Li, J. Shi, H. L. Pan, and M. Li. "Endogenous Anandamide and Cannabinoid Receptor-2 Contribute to Electroacupuncture Analgesia in Rats," *J. Pain* 10:7 (July 2009), 732–39.

Chou, R., J. C. Ballantyne, G. J. Fanciullo, et al. "Research Gaps on Use of Opioids for Chronic Noncancer Pain: Findings from a Review of the Evidence for an American Pain Society and American Academy of Pain Medicine Clinical Practice Guideline," *J. Pain* 10 (2009), 147–59.

Chou, R., R. Deyo, B. Devine, et al. *The Effectiveness and Risks of Long-Term Opioid Treatment of Chronic Pain.* Rockville, MD: Agency for Healthcare Research and Quality, 2014, www .ncbi.nlm.nih.gov/books/NBK258809.

Cichewicz, D. L., and S. P. Welch. "Modulation of Oral Morphine Antinociceptive Tolerance and Naloxone-Precipitated Withdrawal Signs by Oral Delta 9-Tetrahydrocannabinol," *J. Pharmacol. Exp. Ther.* 305:3 (June 2003), 812–17.

Clapper, J. R., G. Moreno-Sanz, R. Russo, et al. "Anandamide Suppresses Pain Initiation through a Peripheral Endocannabinoid Mechanism," *Nature Neuroscience* 13:10 (2010), 1265–70.

Cocteau, Jean. *Opium.* London: Peter Owens Publishers, 1930.

Collen, M. "Prescribing Cannabis for Harm Reduction," *Harm Reduction Journal* 9 (2012), 1.

Compton, Wilson M., Christopher M. Jones, and Grant T. Baldwin. "Relationship between Nonmedical Prescription-Opioid Use and Heroin Use," *New England Journal of Medicine* 374 (2016), 154–63.

Cone, E. J., R. E Johnson, J. D. Moore, and J. D. Roache. "Acute Effects of Smoking Marijuana on Hormones, Subjective Effects and Performance in Male Human Subjects," *Pharmacol. Biochem. Behav.* 24:6 (1986), 1749–54.

Conrad, C., H. M. Bradley, D. Broz, et al. "Community Outbreak of HIV Infection Linked to Injection Drug Use of Oxymorphone, Indiana, 2015," *Morbidity and Mortality Weekly Report* 64:16 (2015), 443–4.

Conte, A., C. M. Bettolo, E. Onesti, V. Frasca, E. Iacovelli, F. Gilio, E. Giacomelli, et al. "Cannabinoid-Induced Effects on the Nociceptive System: A Neurophysiological Study in Patients with Secondary Progressive Multiple Sclerosis," *Eur. J. Pain* 13:5 (May 2009), 472–77.

Cooper, Z. D., S. D. Comer, and M. Haney. "Comparison of the Analgesic Effects of Dronabinol and Smoked Marijuana in Daily Marijuana Smokers," *Neuropsychopharmacology* 38:10 (2013), 1984–92.

Corless, I. B., T. Lindgren, W. Holzemer, L. Robinson, S. Moezzi, K. Kirksey, C. Coleman, et al. "Marijuana Effectiveness as an HIV Self-Care Strategy," *Clin. Nurs. Res.* 18:2 (May 2009), 172–93.

Corroon, J. M. Jr., L. K. Mischley, and M. Sexton. "Cannabis as a Substitute for Prescription Drugs: A Cross-sectional Study," *J. Pain. Res.* 10 (May 2, 2017), 989–98.

Costa, B., A. E. Trovato, F. Comelli, G. Giagnoni, and M. Colleoni. "The Nonpsychoactive Cannabis Constituent Cannabidiol Is an Orally Effective Therapeutic Agent in Rat Chronic Inflammatory and Neuropathic Pain," *Eur. J. Pharmacol.* 556:1–3 (2007), 75–83.

Costa, B., G. Giagnoni, C. Franke, A. E. Trovato, and M. Colleoni. "Vanilloid TRPV1 Receptor Mediates the Antihyperalgesic Effect of the Nonpsychoactive Cannabinoid, Cannabidiol, in a Rat Model of Acute Inflammation," *British Journal of Pharmacology* 143:2 (2004), 247–50.

Costiniuk, C. T., E. Mills, and C. L. Cooper. "Evaluation of Oral Cannabinoid-Containing Medications for the Management of Interferon and Ribavirin-Induced Anorexia, Nausea and Weight Loss in Patients Treated for Chronic Hepatitis C Virus," *Can. J. Gastroenterol.* 22:4 (April 2008), 376–80.

Cottler, L. B., W. M. Compton III, D. Mager, E. L. Spitznagel, and A. Janca. "Posttraumatic Stress Disorder among Substance Users from the General Population," *Am. J. Psychiatry* 149:5 (May 1992), 664–70.

Cox, M. L., V. L. Haller, and S. P. Welch. "Synergy between Delta9-Tetrahydrocannabinol and Morphine in the Arthritic Rat," *Eur. J. Pharmacol.* 567:1–2 (July 12, 2007), 125–30.

Craig, B. W., R. Brown, and J. Everhart. "Effects of Progressive Resistance Training on Growth Hormone and Testosterone Levels in Young and Elderly Subjects," *Mech. Ageing Dev.* 49:2 (August 1989), 159–69.

Cravatt, Benjamin F., Kristin Demarest, Matthew P. Patricelli, Michael H. Bracey, Dan K. Giang, Billy R. Martin, and Aron H. Lichtman. "Supersensitivity to Anandamide and Enhanced Endogenous Cannabinoid Signaling in Mice Lacking Fatty Acid Amide Hydrolase, *PNAS* 98:16, 9371–76.

Creswell, J. D., M. R. Irwin, L. J. Burklund, et al. "Mindfulness-Based Stress Reduction Training Reduces Loneliness and Pro-Inflammatory Gene Expression in Older Adults: A Small Randomized Controlled Trial," *Brain, Behavior, and Immunity* 26:7 (2012), 1095–110.

Crippa, J. A., A. W. Zuardi, and J. E. Hallak. "Therapeutical Use of the Cannabinoids in Psychiatry," *Rev. Bras. Psiquiatr.* 32 (May 2010), suppl. 1, S56–66.

Crippa, J. A., A. W. Zuardi, R. Martín-Santos, S. Bhattacharyya, Z. Atakan, P. McGuire, and P. Fusar-Poli. "Cannabis and Anxiety: A Critical Review of the Evidence," *Hum. Psychopharmacol.* 24:7 (October 2009), 515–23.

Crumpe, S., S. An Inquiry into the Nature and Properties of Opium: Wherein Its Component Principles, Mode of Operation, and Use or Abuse in Particular Diseases, Are Experimentally Investigated, and the Opinions of Former Authors on These Points Impartially Examined London: G. G. and J. Robinson, 1793.

da Silva Torres, I. L., S. N. Cucco, M. Bassani, M. S. Duarte, P. P. Silveira, A. P. Vasconcellos, A. S. Tabajara, et al. "Long-lasting Delayed Hyperalgesia after Chronic Restraint Stress in Rats: Effect Of Morphine Administration," *Neurosci. Res.* 45:3 (2003), 277–83.

Daniell, H. W. "Opioid Endocrinopathy in Women Consuming Prescribed Sustained-Action Opioids for Control of Nonmalignant Pain," *J. Pain* 9 (2008), 28–36.

Dary, David. *Frontier Medicine* (New York: Alfred Knopf, 2008), 36.

De Laurentiis, A., J. Fernández-Solari, C. Mohn, M. Zorrilla Zubilete, and V. Rettori. "Endocannabinoid System Participates in Neuroendocrine Control of Homeostasis," *Neuroimmunomodulation* 17:3 (2010), 153–56.

De Petrocellis, L., A. Ligresti, A. S. Moriello, et al. "Effects of Cannabinoids and Cannabinoid-Enriched Cannabis Extracts on TRP Channels and Endocannabinoid Metabolic Enzymes," *British Journal of Pharmacology* 163:7 (2011), 1479–94.

Dejesus, E., B. M. Rodwick, D. Bowers, C. J. Cohen, and D. Pearce. "Use of Dronabinol Improves Appetite and Reverses Weight Loss in HIV/ AIDS-Infected Patients," *J. Int. Assoc. Physicians AIDS Care* 6:2 (2007), 95–100.

Del Arco, I., M. Navarro, A. Bilbao, B. Ferrer, D. Piomelli, and F. Rodríguez De Fonseca. "Attenuation of Spontaneous Opiate Withdrawal in Mice by the Anandamide Transport Inhibitor AM404. *Eur. J. Pharmacol.* 454:1 (November 1, 2002), 103–4.

DeMause, Lloyd. *Emotional Life of Nations.* New York: Karnac, 2002, http://psychohistory.com/books/the-emotional-life-of-nations.

Dembiński, A., Z. Warzecha, P. Ceranowicz, A. M. Warzecha, W. W. Pawlik, M. Dembiński, K. Rembiasz, et al. "Dual, Time-Dependent Deleterious and Protective Effect of Anandamide on the Course of Cerulein-Induced Acute Pancreatitis: Role of Sensory Nerves," *Eur. J. Pharmacol.* 591:1–3 (September 4, 2008), 284–92.

Devane, W. A., F. A. Dysarz III, M. R. Johnson, L. S. Melvin, and A. C. Howlett. "Determination and Characterization of a Cannabinoid Receptor in Rat Brain," *Mol. Pharmacol.* 34:5 (November 1988), 605–13.

Devane, W. A., L. Hanus, A. Breuer, R. G. Pertwee, L. A. Stevenson, G. Griffin, D. Gibson, A. Mandelbaum, A. Etinger, and R. Mechoulam. "Isolation and Structure of a Brain Constituent that Binds to the Cannabinoid Receptor," *Science* 258 (1992), 1946–49.

Dhalla, I. A., T. Gomes, M. M. Mamdani, and D. N. Juurlink. "Opioids versus Nonsteroidal Anti-Inflammatory Drugs in NonCancer Pain," *Canadian Family Physician* 58:1 (2012), 30.

Dikötter, F., L. Laaman, and Z. Xun. *Narcotic Culture: A History of Drugs in China*. Chicago: University of Chicago Press, 2004.

Dogrul, A., M. Seyrek, B. Yalcin, and A. Ulugol. "Involvement of Descending Serotonergic and Noradrenergic Pathways in CB1 Receptor-Mediated Antinociception," *Prog. Neuropsychopharmacol. Biol. Psychiatry* 38 (2012), 97–105.

Dorsey, John M., ed. *The Jefferson-Dunglison Letters*. Charlottesville, VA: University of Virginia Press, 1960.

Dreborg, Susanne, Görel Sundström, Tomas A. Larsson, and Dan Larhammar. "Evolution of Vertebrate Opioid Receptors," *PNAS* 105:40, 15487–92.

Dreser, Heinrich. "Heroin: A New Derivative of Morphine," *Le Bul. Méd.* 80 (October 5, 1898).

DrugBank Database. "Carfentanil," www.drugbank.ca/drugs/DB01535.

Dufton, L. M., B. Konik, R. Colletti, C. Stanger, M. Boyer, S. Morrow, B. E. Compas. "Effects of Stress on Pain Threshold and Tolerance in Children with Recurrent Abdominal Pain," *Pain* 136:1–2 (2008), 38–43.

Durst, Ronen, Haim Danenberg, Ruth Gallily, Raphael Mechoulam, Keren Meir, Etty Grad, Ronen Beeri, et al. "Cannabidiol, a Nonpsychoactive Cannabis Constituent, Protects against Myocardial Ischemic Reperfusion Injury," *Am. J. Physiol. Heart Circ. Physiol.* 293 (2007), H3602–7.

Dyson, A., M. Peacock, A. Chen, J. P. Courade, M. Yaqoob, A. Groarke, C. Brain, et al. "Antihyperalgesic Properties of the Cannabinoid CT-3 in Chronic Neuropathic and Inflammatory Pain States in the Rat," *Pain* 116:1–2 (July 2005), 129–37.

Ehrlich, I., Y. Humeau, F. Grenier, S. Ciocchi, C. Herry, and A. Lüthi. "Amygdala Inhibitory Circuits and the Control of Fear Memory," *Neuron* 62:6 (June 25, 2009), 757–71.

El-Alfy, Abir T., Kelly Ivey, Keisha Robinson, Safwat Ahmed, Mohamed Radwan, Desmond Slade, Ikhlas Khan, et al. "Antidepressant-like Effect of Δ9-Tetrahydrocannabinol and Other Cannabinoids Isolated from *Cannabis sativa* L.," *Pharmacology Biochemistry and Behavior* 95:4 (June 2010), 434–42.

El-Mallakh, R. S., and C. Brown. "The Effect of Extreme Marijuana Use on the Long-Term Course of Bipolar I Illness: A Single Case Study," *J. Psychoactive Drugs* 39:2 (2007), 201–2.

Elias, A. N., S. Guich, and A. F. Wilson. "Ketosis with Enhanced GABAergic Tone Promotes Physiological Changes in Transcendental Meditation," *Elsevier* 54:4 (April 2000), 660–62.

Ellis, R. J., W. Topero, F. Vaida, G. van den Brande, J. Gonzales, B. Gouaux, H. Bentley, and J. H. Atkinson. "Smoked Medicinal Cannabis for Neuropathic Pain in HIV: A Randomized, Crossover Clinical Trial," *Neuro-psychopharmacology* 34:3 (February 2009), 672–80.

European Medicines Agency. "The European Medicines Agency Recommends Suspension of the Marketing Authorisation of Acomplia," October 23, 2008. Doc. ref. EMEA/CHMP/537777/2008.

———. "Medicinal Product No Longer Authorized: Acomplia (rimonabant)," January 30, 2009, http://goo.gl/yB6tu1.

European Monitoring Centre for Drugs and Drug Addiction. "Fentanyl Drug Profile," www.emcdda.europa.eu/publications/drug-profiles/fentanyl#pharmacology.

———. "Portugal: Country Drug Report," 2017, doi:10.2810/457245.

Fareed, A., P. Eilender, M. Haber, J. Bremner, N. Whitfield, and K. Drexler. "Comorbid Post-traumatic Stress Disorder and Opiate Addiction: A Literature Review," *J. Addict. Dis.* 32:2 (2013), 168–79.

Farquhar-Smith, William P., M. Egertová, E. J. Bradbury, S. B. McMahon, A. S. Rice, and M. R. Elphick. "Cannabinoid CB(1) Receptor Expression in Rat Spinal Cord," *Mol. Cell. Neurosci*15 (2000), 510–21.

Farquhar-Smith, William P. "Peripheral Cannabinoid Analgesia: Neuronal and Immune Mechanisms," *Reviews in Analgesia* 8:2 (2005), 103–16.

Feinberg, I., R. Jones, J. M. Walker, C. Cavness, and J. March. "Effects of High Dosage Delta-9-Tetrahydrocannabinol on Sleep Patterns in Man," *Clin. Pharmacol. Ther.* 17:4 (April 1975), 458–66.

Feinberg, I., R. Jones, J. M. Walker, C. Cavness, and T. Floyd. "Effects of Marijuana Extract and Tetrahydrocannabinol on Electroencephalographic Sleep Patterns," *Clin. Pharmacol. Ther.* 19:6 (June 1976), 782–94.

Felder, C. C., K. E. Joyce, E. M. Briley, J. Mansouri, K. Mackie, O. Blond, Y. Lai, A. L. Ma, and R.L. Mitchell. "Comparison of the Pharmacology and Signal Transduction of the Human Cannabinoid CB1 and CB2 Receptors," *Mol. Pharmacol.* 48:3 (September 1995), 443–50.

Feng, P., J. J. Meissler Jr., M. W. Adler, and T. K. Eisenstein. "Morphine Withdrawal Sensitizes Mice to Lipopolysaccharide: Elevated TNF-alpha and Nitric Oxide with Decreased IL-12," *J. Neuroimmunol.* 164 (2005), 57–65.

Fernández-Ruiz, J., O. Sagredo, M. R. Pazos, et al. "Cannabidiol for Neurodegenerative Disorders: Important New Clinical Applications for This Phytocannabinoid?" *British Journal of Clinical Pharmacology* 75:2 (2013), 323–33.

Fernandez-Solari, J., J. P. Prestifilippo, P. Vissio, M. Ehrhart-Bornstein, S. R. Bornstein, V. Rettori, and J. C. Elverdin. "Anandamide Injected into the Lateral Ventricle of the Brain Inhibits Submandibular Salivary Secretion by Attenuating Parasympathetic Neurotransmission," *Braz. J. Med. Biol. Res.* 42:6 (June 2009), 537–44.

Feuerstein, T. J., O. Gleichauf, D. Peckys, G. B. Landwehrmeyer, R. Scheremet, and R. Jackisch. "Opioid Receptor-Mediated Control of Acetylcholine Release in Human Neocortex Tissue" *Naunyn-Schmiedeberg's Arch. Pharmacol.* 354 (2000), 586–92.

Finnerup, N. B., N. Attal, S. Haroutounian, et al. "Pharmacotherapy for Neuropathic Pain in Adults: Systematic Review, Meta-Analysis and Updated NeuPSIG Recommendations," *The Lancet Neurology* 14:2 (2015), 162–73.

Flor, H., T. Fydrich, and D. C. Turk. "Efficacy of Multidisciplinary Pain Treatment Centers: A Meta-analytic Review," *Pain* 49 (1992), 221–30.

Fournier, G., C. Richez-Dumanois, J. Duvezin, J.-P. Mathieu, and M. Paris. "Identification of a New Chemotype in *Cannabis sativa:* Cannabigerol-Dominant Plants, Biogenetic and Agronomic Prospects," *Plant. Med.* 53 (1987), 277–80.

Frederickson, R. C., C. R. Hewes, and J. W. Aiken. "Correlation between the In Vivo and an In Vitro Expression of Opiate Withdrawal Precipitated by Naloxone: Their Antagonism by l-(-)-Delta9-Tetrahydrocannabinol," *J. Pharmacol. Exp. Ther.* 199:2 (November 1976), 375–84.

Friedrich, G., W. Nepita, and T. Andre. "Serum Testosterone Concentrations in Cannabis and Opiate Users," *Beitr. Gerichtl. Med.* 48 (1990), 57–66.

Fujimori, M., and H. E. Himwich. "Delta 9-Tetrahydrocannabinol and the Sleep-Wakefulness Cycle in Rabbits," *Physiol. Behav.* 11:3 (September 1973), 291–95.

Gabra, Saber. "Papaver Species and Opium through the Ages," *Bulletin de l'Institut d'Egypte* 1956, 40.

Galeni, Claudii. *Medicorum Graecorum opera quae exstant* (Leipzig: B. G. Teubner, 1826), vol. XIII, 273.

Gallily, R., Z. Yekhtin, and L. O. Hanuš. "Overcoming the Bell-Shaped Dose-Response of Cannabidiol by Using Cannabis Extract Enriched in Cannabidiol," *Pharmacology & Pharmacy* 6 (2015), 75–85.

Gaoni, Y., and R. Mechoulam. "Isolation, Structure and Partial Synthesis of an Active Constituent of Hashish," *J. Am. Chem. Soc.* 86:620 (1964), 1646–47.

Gardner, E. "Endocannabinoid Signaling System and Brain Reward: Emphasis on Dopamine," *Pharmacol. Biochem. Behav.* 81 (2005), 263–84.

Gaskell, H., S. Derry, R. A. Moore, H. J. McQuay. "Single-Dose Oral Oxycodone and Oxycodone Plus Paracetamol (Acetaminophen) for Acute Postoperative Pain in Adults," *Cochrane Database Syst. Rev.* 2009:3, CD002763.

Gasser, P., D. Holstein, and Y. Michel. "Safety and Efficacy of Lysergic Acid Diethylamide-Assisted Psychotherapy for Anxiety Associated with Life-Threatening Diseases," *Journal Nerv. Ment. Dis.* 202 (2014), 513–20.

Gatchel, R. J., C. E. Noe, N. M. Garaj, A. S. Vakharia, P. B. Polatin, M. Dreschner, and C. Pulliam. "Treatment carve-out practices: their effect on managing pain at an interdisciplinary pain center," *J. Work. Comp.* 10 (2001), 50–63.

Gazyakan, E., M. Hennegriff, A. Haaf, G. B. Landwehrmeyer, T. J Feuerstein, and R. Jackisch. "Characterization of Opioid Receptor Types Modulating Acetylcholine Release in Septal Regions of the Rat Brain," *Naunyn-Schmiedeberg's Arch Pharmacol.* 362 (2000), 32–40.

Genaro, K., D. Fabris, A. L. F. Arantes, A. W. Zuardi, J. A. S. Crippa, and W. A. Prado. "Cannabidiol Is a Potential Therapeutic for the Affective-Motivational Dimension of Incision Pain in Rats," *Frontiers in Pharmacology* 8 (2017), 391.

Gertsch, J., M. Leonti, S. Raduner, et al. "Beta-Caryophyllene Is a Dietary Cannabinoid," *Proceedings of the National Academy of Sciences of the USA* 105:26 (2008), 9099–104.

Gibran, Khalil. "On Pain." In *The Prophet*. New York: Knopf, 1929.

Glick, S. D., and I. S. Maisonneuve. "Mechanisms of Antiaddictive Actions of Ibogaine," *Ann. NY Acad. Sci.* 844 (1998), 214–26.

Global Biodiversity Information Facility, GBIF Backbone Taxonomy. "*Papaver somniferum* L.," Sp. pl. 1:508. http://doi.org/10.15468/39omei. Accessed August 21, 2017.

Gold, M. S., A. L. Pottash, and I. Extein. "Clonidine: Inpatient Studies from 1978 to 1981," *J. Clin. Psychiatry* 43 (1982), 35–8.

Gold, M. S., D. E. Redmond Jr., and H. D. Kleber. "Noradrenergic Hyperactivity in Opiate Withdrawal Supported by Clonidine Reversal of Opiate Withdrawal," *Am. J. Psychiatry* 136 (1979), 100–2.

Gómez, R., M. Navarro, B. Ferrer, J. M. Trigo, A. Bilbao, I. Del Arco, A. Cippitelli, et al. "A Peripheral Mechanism for CB1 Cannabinoid Receptor-Dependent Modulation of Feeding," *J. Neurosci.* 22:21 (November 1, 2002), 9612–17.

Gorelick, David A., Robert S. Goodwin, Eugene Schwilke, Jennifer R. Schroeder, David M. Schwope, Deanna L. Kelly, Catherine Ortemann-Renon, et al. "Around-the-Clock Oral THC Effects on Sleep in Male Chronic Daily Cannabis Smokers," *American Journal on Addiction* 22:5 (September–October 2013), 510–14.

Greenwald, Glenn. "Drug Decriminalization in Portugal: Lessons for Creating Fair and Successful Drug Policies," white paper, Cato Institute, 2009.

Griffiths, Roland R., Matthew W. Johnson, Michael A. Carducci, Annie Umbricht, William A. Richards, Brian D. Richards, Mary P. Cosimano, and Margaret A. Klinedinst. "Psilocybin Produces Substantial and Sustained Decreases in Depression and Anxiety in Patients with Life-Threatening Cancer: A Randomized Double-Blind Trial, *Journal of Psychopharmacology* 30:12 (2016).

Grimaldi, P., D. Di Giacomo, R. Geremia. "The Endocannabinoid System and Spermatogenesis," *Frontiers in Endocrinology* 4 (2013), 192.

Grinspoon, L., and J. B. Bakalar. "The Use of Cannabis as a Mood Stabilizer in Bipolar Disorder: Anecdotal Evidence and the Need for Clinical Research," *J. Psychoactive Drugs* 30:2 (April–June 1998), 171–77.

Grob, C. S., A. L. Danforth, and G. S. Chopra. "Pilot Study of Psilocybin Treatment for Anxiety in Patients with Advanced-Stage Cancer, *Arch. Gen. Psychiatry* 68 (2011), 71–78.

Grof, Stanislav. *Beyond the Brain: Birth, Death, and Transcendence in Psychotherapy*. Albany, NY: State University of New York Press, 1985.

———. *Healing Our Deepest Wounds: The Holotropic Paradigm Shift*. Newcastle, WA: Stream of Experience, 2012.

Grossman, M. R., A. K. Berkwitt, R. R. Osborn, Y. Xu, D. A. Esserman, E. D. Shapiro, and M. J. Bizzarro. "An Initiative to Improve the Quality of Care of Infants with Neonatal Abstinence Syndrome," *Pediatrics* pii:e20163360 (May 18, 2017), doi:10.1542/peds.2016-3360.

Gruber, Staci A., Kelly A. Sagar, Mary K. Dahlgren, Megan T. Racine, Rosemary T. Smith, and Scott E. Lukas. "Splendor in the Grass? A Pilot Study Assessing the Impact of Medical Marijuana on Executive Function," *Front. Pharmacol.* 7 (October 13, 2016), 355.

Gruenewald, T. L., M. E. Kemeny, N. Aziz, and J. L. Fahey. "Acute Threat to the Social Self: Shame, Social Self-Esteem, and Cortisol Activity," *Psychosom. Med.* 66:6 (November–December 2004), 915–24.

Gunduz-Cinar, O., K. P. MacPherson, R. Cinar, J. Gamble-George, K. Sugden, B. Williams, et al. "Convergent Translational Evidence of a Role for Anandamide in Amygdala-Mediated Fear Extinction, Threat Processing and Stress-Reactivity," *Mol. Psychiatry* 18 (2013), 813–23.

Gupta, Ravi, Nilay D. Shah, and Joseph S. Ross. "The Rising Price of Naloxone: Risks to Efforts to Stem Overdose Deaths," *New England Journal of Medicine* 375 (2016), 2213–15.

GW Pharmaceuticals. "Epidiolex," www.gwpharm.com/epilepsy-patients-caregivers/patients.

Haj-Dahmane, S., and R. Y. Shen. "Modulation of the Serotonin System by Endocannabinoid Signaling," *Neuropharmacology* 61:3 (September 2011), 414–20.

Hall, H. R. "Notices of Recent Publications," *Journal of Egyptian Archaeology* 14 (1928).

Hamelink, Carol, Aidan Hampson, David A. Wink, Lee E. Eiden, and Robert L. Eskay. "Comparison of Cannabidiol, Antioxidants, and Diuretics in Reversing Binge Ethanol-Induced Neurotoxicity," *JPET* 314:2 (August 2005), 780–88.

Hampson, A. J., M. Grimaldi, J. Axelrod, D. Wink. "Cannabidiol and (–)Δ9-Tetrahydrocannabinol are Neuroprotective Antioxidants," *Proceedings of the National Academy of Sciences of the USA* 95:14 (1998), 8268–73.

Hari, Johann. *Chasing the Scream: The First and Last Days on the War on Drugs.* New York: Bloomsbury, 2015.

———. "Everything You Think You Know about Addiction Is Wrong," TED Talk, June 2015, http://goo.gl/kbcBSX.

Hartley, J. P., S. G. Nogrady, and A. Seaton. "Bronchodilator Effect Of Delta1-Tetrahydrocannabinol," *Br. J. Clin. Pharmacol.* 5:6 (June 1978), 523–25.

Hashibe, M., H. Morgenstern, Y. Cui, D. P. Tashkin, Z. F. Zhang, W. Cozen, T. M. Mack, and S. Greenland. "Marijuana Use and the Risk of Lung and Upper Aerodigestive Tract Cancers: Results of a Population-Based Case-Control Study," *Cancer Epidemiol. Biomarkers Prev.* 15:10 (October 2006), 1829–34.

Hatch, Peter J., and Edwin Morris Betts. *Thomas Jefferson's Flower Garden at Monticello,* 3rd ed. Charlottesville, VA: University of Virginia Press, 1971.

Hausknecht, Kathryn, Samir Haj-Dahmane, and Roh-Yu Shen. "Prenatal Stress Exposure Increases the Excitation of Dopamine Neurons in the Ventral Tegmental Area and Alters Their Reponses to Psychostimulants," *Neuropsychopharmacology* 38 (2013), 293–301.

Hayakawa, K., K. Mishima, K. Abe, N. Hasebe, F. Takamatsu, H. Yasuda, T. Ikeda, et al. "Cannabidiol Prevents Infarction via the Non-CB1 Cannabinoid Receptor Mechanism," *Neuroreport* 15:15 (October 25, 2004), 2381–85.

Hernández, A., M. A. Sola, B. Domínguez, M. I. Rochera, P. Bascuñana, and V. Gancedo. "Is Morphine Still the Analgesic of Choice in Acute Myocardial Infarction?" *Rev. Esp. Anestesiol. Reanim.* 55:1 (January 2008), 32–39.

Hesiod. *Theogony,* 11.535–37.

Heyman, E., F. X. Gamelin, M. Goekint, F. Piscitelli, B. Roelands, E. Leclair, V. Di Marzo, and R. Meeusen. "Intense Exercise Increases Circulating Endocannabinoid and BDNF Levels in Humans—Possible Implications for Reward and Depression," *Psychoneuroendocrinology* 37:6 (June 2012), 844–51.

Hien, D. A., H. Jiang, A. N. C. Campbell, M. C. Hu, G. M. Miele, L. R. Cohen, G. S. Brigham, et al. "Do Treatment Improvements in PTSD Severity Affect Substance Use Outcomes? A Secondary Analysis from a Randomized Clinical Trial in NIDA's Clinical Trials Network," *American Journal of Psychiatry* 167 (2010), 95–101.

High Times. "The Strongest Strains on Earth," *High Times, May 2017. High-performance liquid* chromatography lab testing done by Canna Safe Analytics, Murrieta, CA.

Hill, L. E., S. K. Droste, D. J. Nutt, A. C. Linthorst, and J. M. Reul. "Voluntary Exercise Alters GABA(A) Receptor Subunit and Glutamic Acid Decarboxylase-67 Gene Expression in the Rat Forebrain," *J. Psychopharmacol.* 24:5 (May 2010), 745–56.

Hillig, Karl W., and Paul G. Mahlberg. "A Chemotaxonomic Analysis of Cannabinoid Variation in Cannabis (Cannabaceae)," *Am. J. Bot.* 91:6 (June 2004), 966–75.

Hippocrates. *Œuvres complètes d'Hippocrate.*

Hirokami, M., H. Togashi, M. Matsumoto, M. Yoshioka, and H. Saito. "The Functional Role of Opioid Receptors in Acetylcholine Release in the Rat Adrenal Medulla," *Eur. J. Pharmacol.* 253 (1994), 9–15.

Hoffman, E. M., J. C. Watson, J. St. Sauver, N. P. Staff, and C. J. Klein. "Association of Long-Term Opioid Therapy With Functional Status, Adverse Outcomes, and Mortality Among Patients With Polyneuropathy," *JAMA Neurol.* 74:7 (July 1, 2017), 773–79.

Hohmann, A. G., and J. M. Walker. "Cannabinoid Suppression of Noxious Heat-Evoked Activity in Wide Dynamic Range Neuron in the Lumbar Dorsal Horn of the Rat, *J. Neurophysiol.* 81 (1999), 575–83.

Hornby, Antony Paul. Hayley's Comet. patent CA2737447A1, filed April 27, 2011.

Houser, S. J., M. Eads, J. P. Embrey, and S. P. Welch. "Dynorphin B and Spinal Analgesia: Induction of Antinociception by the Cannabinoids CP55,940, Delta(9)-THC and Anandamide," *Brain Res.* 857: 1–2 (February 28, 2000), 337–42.

Hughes, Caitlin Elizabeth, and Alex Stevens. "A Resounding Success or a Disastrous Failure: Reexamining the Interpretation of Evidence on the Portuguese Decriminalization of Illicit Drugs," *Drug and Alcohol Review* 31:1 (January 2012), 101–13.

———. "What Can We Learn from the Portuguese Decriminalization of Illicit Drugs?" *British Journal of Criminology* 50:6 (November 1, 2010), 999–1022.

Hughes, J., T. W. Smith, H. W. Kosterlitz, L. A. Fothergill, B. A. Morgan, and H. R. Morris. "Identification of Two Related Pentapeptides from the Brain with Potent Opiate Agonist Activity," *Nature* 258:5536 (December 1975), 577–80.

Hurd, Yasmin L., M. Yoon, A. F. Manini, et al. "Early Phase in the Development of Cannabidiol as a Treatment for Addiction: Opioid Relapse Takes Initial Center Stage," *Neurotherapeutics* 12:4 (2015), 807–15.

Hurd, Yasmin L. "Cannabidiol: Swinging the Marijuana Pendulum From 'Weed' to Medication to Treat the Opioid Epidemic," *Trends Neurosci.* 40:3 (March 2017), 124–27.

Institute of Medicine, Committee on Treatment of Posttraumatic Stress. *Treatment of Posttraumatic Stress Disorder: An Assessment of the Evidence.* Washington, DC: National Academies Press, 2008.

Iuvone, T., G. Esposito, D. De Filippis, C. Scuderi, and L. Steardo. "Cannabidiol: A Promising Drug for Neurodegenerative Disorders?" *CNS Neurosci. Ther.* 15:1 (Winter 2009), 65–75.

Jacobsen, L. K., S. M. Southwick, and T. R. Kosten. "Substance Use Disorders in Patients with Posttraumatic Stress Disorder: A Review of the Literature," *American Journal of Psychiatry* 158 (2001), 1184–90.

Jennings, E. M., B. N. Okine, M. Roche, and D. P. Finn. "Stress-Induced Hyperalgesia," *Prog. Neurobiol.* 121 (2014), 1–18.

Jerusalemin Talmud. Tr. Abodah Zarah.

Jhaveri, M. D., D. R. Sagar, S. J. Elmes, D. A. Kendall, and V. Chapman. "Cannabinoid CB2 Receptor-Mediated Anti-nociception in Models of Acute and Chronic Pain," *Mol. Neurobiol.* 36 (2007), 26–35.

Jiang, Wen, Yun Zhang, Lan Xiao, Jamie Van Cleemput, Shao-Ping Ji, Guang Bai, and Xia Zhang. "Cannabinoids Promote Embryonic and Adult Hippocampus Neurogenesis and Produce Anxiolytic- and Antidepressant-like Effects," *J. Clin. Invest.* 115:11 (2005), 3104–16.

Jo, Y. H., Y. J. Chen, S. C. Chua Jr., D. A. Talmage, and L. W. Role. "Integration of Endocannabinoid and Leptin Signaling in an Appetite-Related Neural Circuit," *Neuron* 48:6 (December 22, 2005), 1055–66.

Johannes, C. B., T. K. Le, X. Zhou, J. A. Johnston, and R. H. Dworkin. "The Prevalence of Chronic Pain in United States Adults: Results of an Internet-Based Survey," *Jounal of Pain* 11 (2010), 1230–39.

Johnston, I. N., E. D. Milligan, J. Wieseler-Frank, M. G. Frank, V. Zapata, J. Campisi, S. Langer, et al. "A Role for Proinflammatory Cytokines and Fractalkine in Analgesia, Tolerance, and Subsequent Pain Facilitation Induced by Chronic Intrathecal Morphine," *J. Neurosci.* 24 (2004), 7353–65.

Jones, G., and R. G. Pertwee. "A Metabolic Interaction In Vivo between Cannabidiol and 1-Tetrahydrocannabinol," *Br. J. Pharmacol.* 45:2 (1972), 375–77.

Kalivas, P. W., and N. D. Volkow. "The Neural Basis of Addiction: A Pathology of Motivation and Choice," *American Journal of Psychiatry* 162:8 (August 2005), 1403–13.

Kalso, E., L. Smith, H. J. McQuay, R. A. Moore. "No Pain, No Gain: Clinical Excellence and Scientific Rigour—Lessons Learned from IA Morphine," *Pain* 98 (2002), 269–75.

Kamper, S. J., A. T. Apeldoorn, A. Chiarotto, R. J. Smeets, R. W. Ostelo, J. Guzman, and M. W. van Tulder. "Multidisciplinary Biopsychosocial Rehabilitation for Chronic Low Back Pain: Cochrane Systematic Review and Meta-analysis," *BMJ* 350 (2015), h444.

Karst, M., K. Salim, S. Burstein, I. Conrad, L. Hoy, and U. Schneider. "Analgesic Effect of the Synthetic Cannabinoid CT-3 on Chronic Neuropathic Pain: A Randomized Controlled Trial," *JAMA* 290:13 (October 1, 2003), 1757–62.

Kathmann, M., K. Flau, A. Redmer, C. Tränkle, and E. Schlicker. "Cannabidiol Is an Allosteric Modulator at Mu- and Delta-Opioid Receptors," *Naunyn Schmiedebergs Arch. Pharmacol.* 372:5 (February 2006), 354–61.

Kathuria, S., S. Gaetani, D. Fegley, F. Valino, A. Duranti, A. Tontini, et al. "Modulation of Anxiety through Blockade of Anandamide Hydrolysis," *Nat. Med.* 9 (2003), 76–81.

Katz, D., I. Katz, B. S. Porat-Katz, and Y. Shoenfeld. "Medical Cannabis: Another Piece in the Mosaic of Autoimmunity?" *Clin. Pharmacol. Ther.* 101:2 (February 2017), 230–38.

Katz, N., and N. A. Mazer. "The Impact of Opioids on the Endocrine System," *Clin. J. Pain* 25:2 (2009), 170–75.

Kaur, R., S. R. Ambwani, and S. Singh. "Endocannabinoid System: A Multi-Facet Therapeutic Target," *Curr. Clin. Pharmacol.* 11:2 (2016), 110–17.

Keith, D. R., E. W. Gunderson, M. Haney, R. W. Foltin, and C. L. Hart. "Smoked Marijuana Attenuates Performance and Mood Disruptions During Simulated Night Shift Work," *Drug Alcohol Depend.* 178 (September 1, 2017), 534–43.

Kelschenbach, J., R. A. Barke, and S. Roy. "Morphine Withdrawal Contributes to Th2 Cell Differentiation by Biasing Cells Toward the Th2 Lineage," *J. Immunol.* 175 (2005), 2655–65.

Kendrick, K. M. "The Neurobiology of Social Bonds," *J. Neuroendocrinol.* 16 (2004), 1007–8.

Kennett, G. A., C. T. Dourish, and G. Curzon. "Antidepressant-like Action of 5-HT1A Agonists and Conventional Antidepressants in an Animal Model of Depression," *European Journal of Pharmacology* 134:3 (February 24, 1987), 265–74.

Kentucky Department for Public Health, Division of Maternal and Child Health. "Neonatal Abstinence Syndrome in Kentucky." Data brief, December 2015.

Kessler, R. C. "Posttraumatic Stress Disorder: The Burden to the Individual and to Society," *J. Clin. Psychiatry* 61 (2000) suppl. 5, 4–12, discussion 13.4.

Ketchen, Bethany, Pamela Eilender, and Ayman Fareed. "Comorbid Post Traumatic Stress Disorder, Pain and Opiate Addiction," in Colin R. Martin, Victor R. Preedy, and Vinood B. Patel, *Comprehensive Guide to Post-Traumatic Stress Disorder* (New York: Springer, 2015), 1–21.

Khantzian, E. J. "The Self-Medication Hypothesis of Addictive Disorders: Focus on Heroin and Cocaine Dependence," *American Journal of Psychiatry* 142:11 (1985), 1259–64.

Kienbaum, P., N. Thürauf, M. C. Michel, N. Scherbaum, M. Gastpar, and J. Peters. "Profound Increase in Epinephrine Concentration in Plasma and Cardiovascular Stimulation after

Mu-Opioid Receptor Blockade in Opioid-Addicted Patients During Barbiturate-Induced Anesthesia for Acute Detoxification," *Anesthesiology* 88:5 (May 1998), 1154–61.

Kingwell, Katie. "Analgesics: Pain Control at the Periphery," *Nature Reviews Drug Discovery* 9 (November 2010), 839.

Kirkham, T. C. "Endocannabinoids in the Regulation of Appetite and Body Weight," *Behav. Pharmacol.* 16:5–6 (September 2005), 297–313.

Kish, S., K. Kalasinsky, P. Derkach, et al. "Striatal Dopaminergic and Serotonergic Markers in Human Heroin Users," *Neuropsychopharmacology* 24 (2001), 561–67.

Kjaer, T. W., C. Bertelsen, P. Piccini, D. Brooks, J. Alving, and H. C. Lou. "Increased Dopamine Tone during Meditation-Induced Change of Consciousness," *Brain Res. Cogn. Brain Res.* 13:2 (April 2002), 255–59.

Klein, T. W. "Cannabinoid-Based Drugs as Anti-Inflammatory Therapeutics," *Nat. Rev. Immunol.* 5:5 (May 2005), 400–11.

Kolodny, R. C., W. H. Masters, R. M. Kolodner, and G. Toro. "Depression of Plasma Testosterone Levels after Chronic Intensive Marihuana Use," *N. Engl. J. Med.* 290:16 (1974), 872–74.

Koob, George F. "The Dark Side of Emotion: The Addiction Perspective," *Eur. J. Pharmacol.* 753 (April 15, 2015), 73–87.

Kosfeld, M., M. Heinrichs, P. J. Zak, U. Fischbacher, and E. Fehr. "Oxytocin Increases Trust in Humans," *Nature* 435:7042 (June 2, 2005), 673–76.

Kovacs, G. L., Z. Sarnyai, and G. Szabo. "Oxytocin and Addiction: A Review," *Psychoneuroendocrinology* 23 (1998), 945–62.

Krenn, H., L. K. Daha, W. Oczenski, and R. D. Fitzgerald. "A Case of Cannabinoid Rotation in a Young Woman with Chronic Cystitis," *J. Pain Symptom Manag.* 25:1 (January 2003), 3–4.

Kritikos, P. G., and S. P. Papadaki. "The History of the Poppy and of Opium and Their Expansion in Antiquity in the Eastern Mediterranean Area," United Nations Office on Drugs and Crime *Bulletin* 19:3 (1967), n. 126, www.unodc.org/unodc/en/data-and-analysis/bulletin /bulletin_1967-01-01_3_page004.html.

Ku, Chi-Mei, and Jin-Yuarn Lin. "Anti-inflammatory Effects of 27 Selected Terpenoid Compounds Tested Through Modulating Th1/Th2 Cytokine Secretion Profiles Using Murine Primary Splenocytes," *Food Chemistry* 141:2 (November 15, 2013), 1104–13.

Lamontagne, D., P. Lépicier, C. Lagneux, and J. F. Bouchard. "The Endogenous Cardiac Cannabinoid System: A New Protective Mechanism against Myocardial Ischemia," *Arch. Mal Coeur Vaiss.* 99:3 (March 2006), 242–46.

Lanuti, M., E. Talamonti, M. Maccarrone, V. Chiurchiù. "Activation of GPR55 Receptors Exacerbates oxLDL-Induced Lipid Accumulation and Inflammatory Responses, while Reducing Cholesterol Efflux from Human Macrophages," *PLoS ONE* 10:5 (2015), e0126839.

Lashkarizadeh, M. R., M. Garshasbi, M. Shabani, S. Dabiri, H. Hadavi, and H. Manafi-Anari. "Impact of Opium Addiction on Levels of Pro- and Anti-inflammatory Cytokines after Surgery," *Addiction & Health* 8:1 (2016), 9–15.

Leboyer, Frédérick. *Birth without Violence,* 4th ed. New York: Healing Arts Press, 2009.

Lee, A. S., and S. M. Twigg. "Opioid-Induced Secondary Adrenal Insufficiency Presenting as Hypercalcaemia," *Endocrinology, Diabetes & Metabolism Case Reports* 2015:150035.

Lee, C., S. Ludwig, and D. R. Duerksen. "Low-Serum Cortisol Associated with Opioid Use: Case Report and Review of the Literature," *Endocrinologist* 12 (2002), 5–8.

Lee, M. S. "Molecular Clock Calibrations and Metazoan Divergence Dates," *J. Mol. Evol.* 49 (1999), 385–91.

Leung, Pamela T. M., Erin M. Macdonald, Irfan A. Dhalla, and David N. Juurlink. "A 1980 Letter on the Risk of Opioid Addiction," *New England Journal of Medicine* 376 (June 1, 2017), 2194–95.

Levy, B., L. Paulozzi, K. A. Mack, and C. M. Jones. "Trends in Opioid Analgesic-Prescribing Rates by Specialty, U.S., 2007–2012," *American Journal of Preventive Medicine* 49:3 (September 2015), 409–13.

Lewekel, F. M., D. Koethe, F. Pahlisch, D. Schreiber, C. W. Gerth, B. M. Nol-den, J. Klosterkötter, et al. "S39-02 Antipsychotic Effects of Cannabidiol," *European Psychiatry* 24 (2009), suppl. 1, S207.

Li, S., J. Li, D. H. Epstein, X. Y. Zhang, T. R. Kosten, and L. Lu. "Serum Cortisol Secretion During Heroin Abstinence Is Elevated Only Nocturnally," *American Journal of Drug and Alcohol Abuse* 34:3 (2008), 321–28.

Lichtman, A. H., S. M. Sheikh, H. H. Loh, and B. R. Martin. "Opioid and Cannabinoid Modulation of Precipitated Withdrawal in Delta(9)-Tetrahydrocannabinol and Morphine-Dependent Mice," *J. Pharmacol. Exp. Ther.* 298:3 (September 2001), 1007–14.

Lijffijt, M., K. Hu, and A. C. Swann. "Stress Modulates Illness-Course of Substance Use Disorders: A Translational Review," *Frontiers in Psychiatry* 5 (2014), 83.

Linge, R., L. Jiménez-Sánchez, L. Campa, F. Pilar-Cuéllar, R. Vidal, A. Pazos, A. Adell, and Á. Díaz. "Cannabidiol Induces Rapid-Acting Antidepressant-like Effects and Enhances Cortical 5-HT/Glutamate Neurotransmission: Role of 5-HT1A Receptors," *Neuropharmacology* 103 (April 2016), 16-26.

Lu, Dai, V. Kiran Vemuri, Richard I. Duclos Jr., and Alexandros Makriyannis. "The Cannabinergic System as a Target for Anti-Inflammatory Therapies," *Current Topics in Medicinal Chemistry* 6:13 (July 2006), 1401–26.

Lu, Y., B. C. Akinwumi, Z. Shao, and H. D. Anderson. "Ligand Activation of Cannabinoid Receptors Attenuates Hypertrophy of Neonatal Rat Cardiomyocytes," *J. Cardiovasc. Pharmacol.* 64:5 (November 2014), 420–30.

Luongo, L., K. Starowicz, S. Maione, and V. Di Marzo. "Allodynia Lowering Induced by Cannabinoids and Endocannabinoids (ALICE)," *Pharmacol. Res.* 119 (May 2017), 272–77.

Lynch, M. E., and F. Campbell. "Cannabinoids for Treatment of Chronic Noncancer Pain: A Systematic Review of Randomized Trials," *British Journal of Clinical Pharmacology* 72:5 (2011), 735–44.

Macht, D. I. "The History of Opium and Some of Its Preparation and Alkaloids," *JAMA* 64 (1915), 477–61.

Maeda, T., and S. Kishioka. "PPAR and Pain," *Int. Rev. Neurobiol.* 85 (2009), 165–77.

Magon, N., and S. Kalra. "The Orgasmic History of Oxytocin: Love, Lust, and Labor," *Indian Journal of Endocrinology and Metabolism* 15:suppl. 3 (2011), S156–61.

Maida, V. "The Synthetic Cannabinoid Nabilone Improves Pain and Symptom Management in Cancer Patients," paper presented at the San Antonio Breast Cancer Symposium, December 2006.

Malinowska, B., G. Godlewski, B. Bucher, E. Schlicker. "Cannabinoid CB1 Receptor-Mediated Inhibition of the Neurogenic Vasopressor Response in the Pithed Rat," *Naunyn-Schmiedeberg's Arch Pharmacol.* 356 (1997), 197–202.

Mandolino, G., and A. Carboni. "Potential of Marker Assisted Selection in Hemp Genetic Improvement," *Euphytica* 140 (2004), 107–20.

Manges, M. "A Second Report on Therapeutics of Heroin," *New York Medical Journal* 71, 51.

Manini, A. F., G. Yiannoulos, M. M. Bergamaschi, et al. "Safety and Pharmacokinetics of Oral Cannabidiol When Administered Concomitantly with Intravenous Fentanyl in Humans," *Journal of Addiction Medicine* 9:3 (2015), 204–10.

Manjiani, D., D. B. Paul, S. Kunnumpurath, A. D. Kaye, and N. Vadivelu. "Availability and Utilization of Opioids for Pain Management: Global Issues," *The Ochsner Journal* 14:2 (2014), 208–15.

Mao, J., B. Sung, R. R. Ji, and G. Lim. "Chronic Morphine Induces Down Regulation of Spinal Glutamate Transporters: Implications in Morphine Tolerance and Abnormal Pain Sensitivity," *J. Neurosci.* 22 (2002), 8312–23.

Mao, J., D. D. Price, J. Lu, L. Keniston, and D. J. Mayer. "Two Distinctive Antinociceptive Systems in Rats with Pathological Pain," *Neurosci. Lett.* 280:1 (February 11, 2000), 13–6.

Markos, J. R., H. M. Harris, W. Gul, M. A. ElSohly, and K. J. Sufka. "Effects of Cannabidiol on Morphine Conditioned Place Preference in Mice," *Planta Med.* August 9, 2017.

Mas-Nieto, Magdalena, Blandine Pommier, Eleni T Tzavara, Anne Caneparo, Sophie Da Nascimento, Gérard Le Fur, Bernard P Roques, and Florence Noble. "Reduction of Opioid Dependence by the CB1 Antagonist SR141716A in Mice: Evaluation of the Interest in Pharmacotherapy of Opioid Addiction," *Br. J. Pharmacol.* 132:8 (April 2001), 1809–16.

Matsuda, K., Y. Mikami, K. Takeda, S. Fukuyama, S. Egawa, M. Sunamura, I. Maruyama, and S. Matsuno. "The Cannabinoid 1 Receptor Antagonist, AM251, Prolongs the Survival of Rats with Severe Acute Pancreatitis," *Tohoku J. Exp. Med.* 207:2 (October 2005), 99–107.

McCauley, J. L., T. Killeen, D. F. Gros, K. T. Brady, S. E. Back. "Posttraumatic Stress Disorder and Co-Occurring Substance Use Disorders: Advances in Assessment and Treatment," *Clinical Psychology* 19:3 (2012), 283–304.

McDonald, D. C., K. Carlson, and D. Izrael. "Geographic Variation in Opioid Prescribing in the U.S.," *Journal of Pain* 13:10 (2012), 988–96.

McHugh, D. "GPR18 in Microglia: Implications for the CNS and Endocannabinoid System Signalling," *British Journal of Pharmacology* 167:8 (2012), 1575–82.

McLaughlin, R. J., M. N. Hill, A. C. Morrish, and B. B. Gorzalka. "Local Enhancement of Cannabinoid CB1 Receptor Signaling in the Dorsal Hippocampus Elicits an Antidepressant-like Effect," *Behav. Pharmacol.* 18:5–6 (September 2007), 431–38.

McPartland, J. M., M. Glass, and R. G. Pertwee. "Meta-analysis of Cannabinoid Ligand Binding Affinity and Receptor Distribution: Interspecies Differences," *British Journal of Pharmacology* 152:5 (2007), 583–93.

McPartland, John M., and Patty Pruitt. "Sourcing the Code: Searching for the Evolutionary Origins of Cannabinoid Receptors, Vanilloid Receptors, and Anandamide," *Journal of Cannabis Therapeutics* 2:1 (2002).

Mechoulam, Raphael. "Conversation with Raphael Mechoulam," *Addiction* 102 (2007), 887–93.

Meier, Barry. "In Guilty Plea, OxyContin Maker to Pay $600 Million," *New York Times* Business Day, May 10, 2007, www.nytimes.com/2007/05/10/business/11drug-web.html.

Meier, M. H., A. Caspi, A. Ambler, H. Harrington, R. Houts, R. S. Keefe, K. McDonald, et al. "Persistent Cannabis Users Show Neuropsychological Decline from Childhood to Midlife," *Proc. Natl. Acad. Sci. USA* 109:40 (October 2, 2012), E2657–64.

Mendelson, J. H., J. Ellingboe, J. C. Kuehnle, and N. K. Mello, "Heroin and Naltrexone Effects on Pituitary-Gonadal Hormones in Man: Interaction of Steroid Feedback Effects, Tolerance and Supersensitivity," *J. Pharmacol. Exp. Ther.* 214 (1980), 503–6.

Mendelson, J. H., J. Kuehnle, J. Ellingboe, and T. F. Babor. "Plasma Testosterone Levels Before, During and After Chronic Marihuana Smoking," *N. Engl. J. Med.* 291:20 (1974), 1051–55.

Meng, I. D., B. H. Manning, W. J. Martin, and H. L. Fields. "An Analgesia Circuit Activated by Cannabinoids," *Nature* 395:6700 (September 24, 1998), 381–83.

Merrer, J., Jaj Becker, K. Befort, and B. Kieffer. "Reward Processing by the Opioid System in the Brain," *Physiological Reviews* 89:4 (2009), 1379–12.

Merskey, Harold, and Nikolai Bogduk. *Classification of Chronic Pain: Description of Chronic Pain Syndromes and Definition of Pain Terms.* Seattle: IASP Press, 1994.

Meunier, J. C., C. Mollereau, L. Toll, C. Suaudeau, C. Moisand, P. Alvinerie, J. L. Butour, J. C. Guillemot, P. Ferrara, and B. Monsarrat. "Isolation and Structure of the Endogenous Agonist of Opioid Receptor-Like ORL1 Receptor," *Nature* 377:6549 (October 1995), 532–35.

Mezzacappa, Elizabeth S., E. S. Katkin, and S. N. Palmer. "Epinephrine, Arousal, and Emotion: A New Look at Two-Factor Theory," *Cognition and Emotion* 13:2 (1999), 181–99.

Michalski, Christoph W., Milena Maier, Mert Erkan, Danguole Sauliunaite, Frank Bergmann, Pal Pacher, Sandor Batkai, et al. "Cannabinoids Reduce Markers of Inflammation and Fibrosis in Pancreatic Stellate Cells," *PLoS ONE* 3:2 (2008), e1701.

Mills, K. L., M. Teesson, J. Ross, and L. Peters. "Trauma, PTSD, and Substance Use Disorders: Findings from the Australian National Survey of Mental Health and Well-Being," *Am. J. Psychiatry* 163:4 (April 2006), 652–8.

Minton, Jonathan, Jane Parkinson, James Lewsey, Janet Bouttell, and Gerry McCartney. "Drug Related Deaths in Scotland," Open Science Framework, July 25, 2017, doi:10.17605/OSF .IO/ECBPN.

Mithoefer, M. C., M. T.Wagner, A. T. Mithoefer, L. Jerome, and R. J. Doblin. "Durability of Improvement in Post–Traumatic Stress Disorder Symptoms and Absence of Harmful Effects or Drug Dependency after 3,4-Methylenedioxymethamphetamine-Assisted Psychotherapy: A Prospective Long-Term Follow-up Study," *Psychopharmacol.* 25 (2011), 439–52.

Mizoguchi, K., A. Ishige, Aburada, and T. Tabira. "Chronic Stress Attenuates Glucocorticoid Negative Feedback: Involvement of the Prefrontal Cortex and Hippocampus," *Neuroscience* 119:3 (2003), 887–97.

Molina, P. E. "Opioids and Opiates: Analgesia with Cardiovascular, Haemodynamic and Immune Implications in Critical Illness," *Journal of Internal Medicine* 259 (2006), 138–54.

Monti, Jaime M. "Hypnoticlike Effects of Cannabidiol in the Rat," *Psychopharmacology* 55:3 (January 1977) 263–65.

Moreira, F. A., and J. A. Crippa. "The Psychiatric Side-Effects of Rimonabant," *Rev. Bras. Psiquiatr.* 31:2 (June 2009), 145–53.

Morris, Robert G., Michael TenEyck, J. C. Barnes, and Tomislav V. Kovandzic. "The Effect of Medical Marijuana Laws on Crime: Evidence from State Panel Data, 1990–2006," *PLoS ONE* 9:3, e92816.

Moseley, G. L., T. J. Parsons, and C. Spence. "Visual Distortion of a Limb Modulates the Pain and Swelling Evoked by Movement," *Curr. Biol.* 18:22 (November 2008), R1047–48.

Muhuri, Pradip K., Joseph C. Gfroerer, and M. Christine Davies. "Associations of Nonmedical Pain Reliever Use and Initiation of Heroin Use in the United States," *Center for Behavioral Health Statistics and Quality Data Review,* August 2013, http://goo.gl/T1ydQi.

Multidisciplinary Association for Psychedelic Studies. "FDA Grants Breakthrough Therapy Designation for MDMA-Assisted Psychotherapy for PTSD, Agrees on Special Protocol Assessment for Phase 3 Trials." Press release, August 26, 2017, http://goo.gl/VNrCi1.

Munro, S., K. L. Thomas, and M. Abu-Shaar. "Molecular Characterization of a Peripheral Receptor for Cannabinoids," *Nature* 365 (1993), 61–65.

Murillo-Rodríguez, E., M. Sánchez-Alavez, L. Navarro, D. Martínez-González, R. Drucker-Colín, and O. Prospéro-García. "Anandamide Modulates Sleep and Memory in Rats," *Brain Res.* 812:1–2 (November 23, 1998), 270–74.

Murillo-Rodríguez, Eric, Andrea Sarro-Ramírez, Daniel Sánchez, Stephanie Mijangos-Moreno, Alma Tejeda-Padrón, Alwin Poot-Aké, Khalil Guzmán, et al. "Potential Effects of Cannabidiol as a Wake-Promoting Agent," *Curr. Neuropharmacol.* 12:3 (May 2014), 269–72.

Nalivaiko, E., Y. Ootsuka, and W. W. Blessing. "Activation of 5-HT1A Receptors in the Medullary Raphe Reduces Cardiovascular Changes Elicited by Acute Psychological and Inflammatory Stresses in Rabbits," *Am. J. Physiol. Regul. Integr. Comp. Physiol.* 289:2 (2005), R596–R604.

Napimoga, M. H., B. B. Benatti, F. O. Lima, P. M. Alves, A. C. Campos, D. R. Pena-Dos-Santos, F. P. Severino, F. Q. Cunha, and F. S. Guimarães. "Cannabidiol Decreases Bone Resorption by Inhibiting RANK/RANKL Expression and Pro-inflammatory Cytokines During Experimental Periodontitis in Rats," *Int. Immunopharmacol.* 9:2 (February 2009), 216–22.

Narang, S., D. Gibson, A. D. Wasan, E. L. Ross, E. Michna, S. S. Nedeljkovic, and R. N. Jamison. "Efficacy of Dronabinol as an Adjuvant Treatment for Chronic Pain Patients on Opioid Therapy," *J. Pain* 9:3 (March 2008), 254–64.

National Center for Biotechnology Information. "PubChem Compound Database," CID=62156, http://pubchem.ncbi.nlm.nih.gov/compound/62156. Accessed September 9, 2017.

National Institute on Drug Abuse. "Fentanyl," www.drugabuse.gov/publications/drugfacts/fentanyl.

Neff, G. W., C. B. O'Brien, K. R. Reddy, N. V. Bergasa, A. Regev, E. Molina, R. Amaro, et al. "Preliminary Observation with Dronabinol in Patients with Intractable Pruritus Secondary to Cholestatic Liver Disease," *Am. J. Gastroenterol.* 97:8 (August 2002), 2117–19.

Nelson, K., D. Walsh, P. Deeter, and F. Sheehan. "A Phase II Study Of Delta-9-Tetrahydrocannabinol for Appetite Stimulation in Cancer-Associated Anorexia," *Journal of Palliative Care* 10:1 (1994), 14–18.

Netherland, Julie, and Helena Hansen, White opioids: Pharmaceutical race and the war on drugs that wasn't," *BioSocieties* 12:2 (June 2017), 217–38.

Neumann, I. D. "The Advantage of Social Living: Brain Neuropeptides Mediate the Beneficial Consequences of Sex and Motherhood," *Front. Neuroendocrinol.* 30 (2009), 483–96.

Nicander of Colophon. *Theriaca et Alexipharmaca* (Leipzig: B. G. Teubner, 1856).

Nicholson, Anthony N., Claire Turner, Barbara M. Stone, and Philip J. Robson. "Effect of D-9-Tetrahydrocannabinol and Cannabidiol on Nocturnal Sleep and Early-Morning Behavior in Young Adults," *Journal of Clinical Psychopharmacology* 24:3 (June 2004).

Niederhoffer, N., H. H. Hansen, J. J. Fernandez-Ruiz, and B. Szabo. "Effects of Cannabinoids on Adrenaline Release from Adrenal Medullary Cells," *British Journal of Pharmacology* 134:6 (2001), 1319–27.

Nikolaou, K., D. Kapoukranidou, S. Ndungu, G. Floros, and L. Kovatsi. "Severity of Withdrawal Symptoms, Plasma Oxytocin Levels, and Treatment Outcome in Heroin Users Undergoing Acute Withdrawal," *J. Psychoactive Drugs* 49:3 (July–August 2017), 233–41.

Noble, M., J. R. Treadwell, S. J. Tregear, V. H. Coates, P. J. Wiffen, C. Akafomo, K. M. Schoelles, and R. Chou. "Long-term Opioid Management for Chronic Noncancer Pain," *Cochrane Database of Systematic Reviews* 1 (CD006605:2010), doi:10.1002/14651858.CD006605.pub2.

Notcutt, W., M. Price, A. Miller, et al. "Initial Experiences with Medicinal Extracts of Cannabis for Chronic Pain: Results from 34 'N of 1' Studies," *Anaesthesia* 59 (2004), 440–52.

Nurmikko, T. J., M. G. Serpell, B. Hoggart, et al. "Sativex Successfully Treats Neuropathic Pain Characterised by Allodynia: A Randomised, Doubleblind, Placebo-Controlled Clinical Trial," *Pain* 133 (2007), 210–20.

O'Connell, B. K., D. Gloss, and O. Devinsky. "Cannabinoids in Treatment-Resistant Epilepsy: A Review," *Epilepsy Behav.* 70:pt. B (May 2017), 341–48.

O'Connell, Thomas J., and Ché B. Bou-Matar. "Long-Term Marijuana Users Seeking Medical Cannabis in California (2001–2007): Demographics, Social Characteristics, Patterns of Cannabis and Other Drug Use of 4,117 Applicants," *Harm Reduction Journal* 4:16 (2007).

O'Sullivan, S. E., and D. A. Kendall. "Cannabinoid Activation of Peroxisome Proliferator-Activated Receptors: Potential for Modulation of Inflammatory Disease," *Immunobiology* 215:8 (August 2010), 611–16.

Orens, Adam, Miles Light, Jacob Rowberry, Jeremy Matsen, and Brian Lewandowski. "Marijuana Equivalency in Portion and Dosage: An assessment of physical and pharmacokinetic relationships in marijuana production and consumption in Colorado," Colorado Department of Revenue, August 10, 2015.

Pagano, E., R. Capasso, F. Piscitelli, B. Romano, O. A. Parisi, S. Finizio, A. Lauritano, et al. "An Orally Active Cannabis Extract with High Content in Cannabidiol attenuates Chemically-Induced Intestinal Inflammation and Hypermotility in the Mouse," *Front. Pharmacol.* 4:7 (October 2016), 341.

Palermo, T. M., E. F. Law, J Fales, M. H. Bromberg, T. Jessen-Fiddick, G. Tai. "Internet-Delivered Cognitive-Behavioral Treatment for Adolescents with Chronic Pain and Their Parents: A Randomized Controlled Multicenter Trial, *Pain* 157:1 (2016), 174–85.

Palkovits, M., "The Brain and the Pain: Neurotransmitters and Neuronal Pathways of Pain Perception and Response," *Orv. Hetil.* 141:41 (October 8, 2000), 2231–39.

Pandey, R., K. Mousawy, M. Nagarkatti, and P. Nagarkatti. "Endocannabinoids and Immune Regulation," *Pharmacological Research* 60:2 (2009), 85–92.

Parker, J., F. Atez, R. G. Rossetti, A. Skulas, R. Patel, and R. B. Zurier. "Suppression of Human Macrophage Interleukin-6 by a Nonpsychoactive Cannabinoid Acid," *Rheumatol. Int.* 28:7 (May 2008), 631–35.

Parolaro, D., N. Realini, D. Vigano, C. Guidali, and T. Rubino. "The Endocannabinoid System and Psychiatric Disorders," *Exp. Neurol.* 224:1 (July 2010), 3–14.

Parsadaniantz, S. Melik, C. Rivat, W. Rostene, and A. Reaux-Le Goazigo. "Opioid and Chemokine Receptor Crosstalk: A Promising Target for Pain Therapy?" *Nat. Rev. Neurosci.*16 (2015), 69–78.

Patrick, L. E., E. M. Altmaier, and E. M. Found. "Long-Term Outcomes in Multidisciplinary Treatment of Chronic Low Back Pain: Results of a 13-Year Follow-up," *Spine* 29 (2004), 850–55.

Peirson, A. R., and J. W. Heuchert. "Correlations for Serotonin Levels and Measures of Mood in a Nonclinical Sample," *Psychol. Rep.* 87:3 (December 2000), 707–16.

Pelliccia, A., G. Grassi, A. Romano, and P. Crocchialo. "Treatment with CBD in Oily Solution of Drug-Resistant Paediatric Epilepsies." Paper presented to the Congress on Cannabis and the Cannabinoids, Leiden, The Netherlands, September 9–10, 2005.

Perrine, Daniel M. *The Chemistry of Mind-Altering Drugs*. Washington, DC: American Chemical Society, 1997.

Pert, C. B., and S. H. Snyder. "Opiate Receptor: Demonstration in Nervous Tissue," *Science* 179:4077 (March 1973), 1011–14.

Pertwee, R. G. "Cannabinoid receptors and pain," *Prog. Neurobiol.* 63 (2001), 569–611.

Petzke, F., E. K. Enax-Krumova, and W. Häuser. "Efficacy, Tolerability and Safety of Cannabinoids for Chronic Neuropathic Pain: A Systematic Review of Randomized Controlled Studies. *Schmerz.* 30:1 (February 2016), 62–88.

Phatak, U. P., D. Rojas-Velasquez, A. Porto, and D. S. Pashankar. "Prevalence and Patterns of Marijuana Use in Young Adults with Inflammatory Bowel Disease," *J. Pediatr. Gastroenterol. Nutr.* 64:2 (February 2017), 261–64.

Physician Payments Sunshine Act of 2009, www.congress.gov/bill/111th-congress/senate-bill/301.

Piburn, Sidney. *The Dalai Lama, a Policy of Kindness: An Anthology of Writings by and About the Dalai Lama*. Delhi: Motilal Banarsidass, 1997.

Piper, B. J., R. M. DeKeuster, M. L. Beals, C. M. Cobb, C. A. Burchman, L. Perkinson, S. T. Lynn, et al. "Substitution of Medical Cannabis for Pharmaceutical Agents for Pain, Anxiety, and Sleep," *J. Psychopharmacol.* 31:5 (May 2017), 569–75.

Plasse, T. F., R. W. Gorter, S. H. Krasnow, M. Lane, K. V. Shepard, and R. G. Wadleigh. "Recent Clinical Experience with Dronabinol," *Pharmacol. Biochem. Behav.* 40:3 (November 1991), 695–700.

Popova, N. K., et al. "Involvement of the 5-HT1A and 5-HT1B Serotonergic Receptor Subtypes in Sexual Arousal in Male Mice," *Psychoneuroendocrinology* 27:5 (July 2002), 609–18.

Portenoy, R. K., and K. M. Foley. "Chronic Use of Opioid Analgesics in Nonmalignant Pain: Report of 38 Cases," *Pain* 25:2 (May 1986), 171–86.

Portenoy, Russell K., Elena Doina Ganae-Motan, Silvia Allende, Ronald Yanagihara, Lauren Shaiova, Sharon Weinstein, Robert McQuade, et al. "Nabiximols for Opioid-Treated Cancer Patients With Poorly-Controlled Chronic Pain: A Randomized, Placebo-Controlled, Graded-Dose Trial," *Journal of Pain* 13:5 (May 2012), 438–49.

ProCon.org. "Deaths from Marijuana v. 17 FDA-Approved Drugs: Jan. 1, 1997 to June 30, 2005," July 8, 2009, http://goo.gl/ygFFby.

PubChem Compound Database. "Carfentanil," http://pubchem.ncbi.nlm.nih.gov/compound/62156. Accessed September 13, 2017.

Quintero, L., M. Moreno, C. Avila, J. Arcaya, W. Maixner, and H. Suarez-Roca. "Long-lasting Delayed Hyperalgesia after Subchronic Swim Stress," *Pharmacol. Biochem. Behav.* 67:3 (2000), 449–58.

Raft, D., J. Gregg, J. Ghia, and L. Harris. "Effects of Intravenous Tetrahydrocannabinol on Experimental and Surgical Pain: Psychological Correlates of the Analgesic Response," *Clin. Pharmacol. Ther.* 21 (1977), 26–33.

Raichlen, D. A., A. D. Foster, G. L. Gerdeman, A. Seillier, and A. Giu Rida. "Wired to Run: Exercise-Induced Endocannabinoid Signaling in Humans and Cursorial Mammals with Implications for the 'Runner's High.'" *J. Exp. Biol.* 215 (April 15, 2012), 1331–36.

Ramachandran, R., E. Hyun, L. Zhao, T. K. Lapointe, K. Chapman, C. L. Hirota, S. Ghosh, et al. "TRPM8 Activation Attenuates Inflammatory Responses in Mouse Models of Colitis," *Proc. Natl. Acad. Sci. USA* 110 (2013), 7476–81.

Reiman, Amanda, Mark Welty, and Perry Solomon. "Cannabis as a Substitute for Opioid-Based Pain Medication: Patient Self-Report," *Cannabis and Cannabinoid Research* 2:1 (June 2017), 160-166.

Resstel, L. B., R. F. Tavares, S. F. Lisboa, S. R. Joca, F. M. Corrêa, and F. S. Guimarães. "5-HT1A Receptors Are Involved in the Cannabidiol-Induced Attenuation of Behavioural and Cardiovascular Responses to Acute Restraint Stress in Rats," *Br. J. Pharmacol.* 156:1 (January 2009), 181–88.

Richardson, D., R. G. Pearson, N. Kurian, et al. "Characterisation of the Cannabinoid Receptor System in Synovial Tissue and Fluid in Patients with Osteoarthritis and Rheumatoid Arthritis," *Arthritis Res. Ther.* 10 (2008), R43.

Riley, J. L., B. A. Hastie, T. L. Glover, C. M. Campbell, R. Staud, R. B. Fillingim. "Cognitive-Affective and Somatic Side Effects of Morphine and Pentazocine: Side-Effect Profiles in Healthy Adults," *Pain Medicine* 11:2 (2010), 10.

Rivers, Jack Rocky-Jay, and John Clive Ashton. "The Development of Cannabinoid CBII Receptor Agonists for the Treatment of Central Neuropathies," *Central Nervous System Agents in Medicinal Chemistry* 10 (2010), 47–64.

Robbins, H., R. J. Gatchel, C. Noe, N. Gajraj, P. Polatin, M. Deschner, A. Vakharia, and L. Adams. "A Prospective One-Year Outcome Study of Interdisciplinary Chronic Pain Management: Compromising Its Efficacy by Managed Care Policies," *Anesthesia & Analgesia* 97 (2003), 156–62.

Roberts, A. H., R. A. Sternbach, and J. Polich. "Behavioral Management of Chronic Pain and Excess Disability: Long-Term Follow-up of an Outpatient Program," *Clin. J. Pain* 9 (1993), 41–48.

Robins, Lee N., John E. Helzer, Michie Hesselbrock, and Eric Wish. "Three Years after Vietnam: How Our Study Changed Our View of Heroin," *The American Journal on Addictions* 19, 203–11.

Robiquet, P.-J. "Nouvelles observations sur les principaux produits de l'opium," *Ann. Chim. Phys.* 51:2 (1832), 225–67.

Rog, D. J., T. Nurmiko, T. Friede, et al. "Randomized Controlled Trial of Cannabis-Based Medicine in Central Neuropathic Pain Due to Multiple Sclerosis," *Neurology* 65 (2005), 812–19.

Room, R. "Stigma, Social Inequality, and Alcohol and Drug Use," *Drug and Alcohol Review* 24 (2005), 143–55.

Rosenthaler, Sarah, Birgit Pöhn, Caroline Kolmanz, Chi Nguyen Huu, Christopher Krewenka, Alexandra Huber, Barbara Kranner, Wolf-Dieter Rausch, and Rudolf Moldzio. "Differences in Receptor Binding Affinity of Several Phytocannabinoids Do Not Explain Their Effects on Neural Cell Cultures," *Neurotoxicology and Teratology* 46 (2014), 49–56.

Rossato, M., F. Ion Popa, M. Ferigo, G. Clari, and C. Foresta. "Human Sperm Express Cannabinoid Receptor Cb1, the Activation of Which Inhibits Motility, Acrosome Reaction, and Mitochondrial Function," *J. Clin. Endocrinol. Metab.* 90:2 (2005), 984–91.

Rubino, T., P. Massi, D. Viganò, D. Fuzio, and D. Parolaro. "Long-Term Treatment with SR141716A, the CB1 Receptor Antagonist, Influences Morphine Withdrawal Syndrome," *Life Sci.* 66:22 (April 21, 2000), 2213–19.

Russo, E. B. "Taming THC: Potential Cannabis Synergy and Phytocannabinoid-Terpenoid Entourage Effects," *British Journal of Pharmacology* 163:7 (2011), 1344–64.

Russo, E. B., and G. W. Guy. "A Tale of Two Cannabinoids: The Therapeutic Rationale for Combining Tetrahydrocannabinol and Cannabidiol," *Med. Hypotheses* 66 (2006), 234–46.

Rydén, Gunnar, and Ingvar Sjöholm. "Half-Life of Oxytocin in Blood of Pregnant and Non-Pregnant Woman," *Acta Obstetricia et Gynecologica Scandinavica* 48: suppl. 3 (1969).

Salimpoor, V. N., M. Benovoy, K. Larcher, A. Dagher, and R. J. Zatorre. "Anatomically Distinct Dopamine Release during Anticipation and Experience of Peak Emotion to Music," *Nat. Neurosci.* 14:2 (February 2011), 257–62.

San Francisco Medical Examiner's Office. *Annual Report, July 1, 1998–June 30, 1999,* 1999:65.

Sarnyai, Z., and G. L. Kovács. "Oxytocin in Learning and Addiction: From Early Discoveries to the Present," *Pharmacol. Biochem. Behav.* 119 (2014), 3–9.

———. "Role of Oxytocin in the Neuroadaptation to Drugs of Abuse," *Psychoneuroendocrinology* 19 (1994), 85–117.

Sartim, A. G., F. S. Guimarães, and S. R. Joca. "Antidepressant-like Effect of Cannabidiol Injection into the Ventral Medial Prefrontal Cortex-Possible Involvement of 5-HT1A and CB1 Receptors," *Behav. Brain Res.* 303 (April 15, 2016), 218–27.

Scavone, J. L., R. C. Sterling, E. J. Van Bockstaele. "Cannabinoid and Opioid Interactions: Implications for Opiate Dependence and Withdrawal," *Neuroscience* 248 (2013), 637–54.

Schaefert, R., P. Welsch, P. Klose, C. Sommer, F. Petzke, and W. Häuser. "Opioids in Chronic Osteoarthritis Pain: A Systematic Review and Meta-analysis of Efficacy, Tolerability and Safety in Randomized Placebo-Controlled Studies of at Least 4 Weeks Duration," *Schmerz.* 29:1 (February 2015), 47–59.

Schneider, Johann Gottlob. *Orpheus' Argonautica,* 1803, 11.914–15.

Schubart, Christian D., et al. "Cannabis with High Cannabidiol Content Is Associated with Fewer Psychotic Experiences," *Schizophrenia Research* 130:1, 216–21.

Seal, K. H., A. H. Kral, L. Gee, L. D. Moore, R. N. Bluthenthal, J. Lorvick, and B. R. Edlin. "Predictors and Prevention of Nonfatal Overdose Among Street-Recruited Injection Heroin

Users in the San Francisco Bay Area, 1998–1999," *American Journal of Public Health* 91:11 (2001), 1842–46.

Secades-Villa, R., O. Garcia-Rodríguez, C. J. Jin, S. Wang, and C. Blanco. "Probability and Predictors of the Cannabis Gateway Effect: A National Study," *International Journal of Drug Policy* 26:2 (2015), 135–42.

Secretary-General of the United Nations. Single Convention on Narcotic Drugs (of 1961). No. 14152. Signed March 30, 1961. In force August 8, 1975. Parties: 185.

Seely, K. A., L. K. Brents, L. N. Franks, M. Rajasekaran, S. M. Zimmerman, W. E. Fantegrossi, P. L. Prather. "AM-251 and Rimonabant Act as Direct Antagonists at Mu-Opioid Receptors: Implications for Opioid/Cannabinoid Interaction Studies." *Neuropharmacology* 63 (2012), 905–15.

Sertürner, F. W. "Über das Morphium, eine neue salzfähige Grundlage, und die Mekonsäure, als Hauptbestandteile des Opiums," *Annalen der Physik* 25 (1817), 56–90.

Shamran, H., N. P. Singh, E. E. Zumbrun, A. Murphy, D. D. Taub, M. K. Mishra, R. L. Price, et al. "Fatty Acid Amide Hydrolase (FAAH) Blockade Ameliorates Experimental Colitis by Altering MicroRNA Expression and Suppressing Inflammation," *Brain Behav. Immun.* 59 (January 2017), 10–20.

Shannon, S., and J. Opila-Lehman. "Effectiveness of Cannabidiol Oil for Pediatric Anxiety and Insomnia as Part of Posttraumatic Stress Disorder: A Case Report," *Perm. J.* 20:4 (Fall 2016), 108–11.

Shin, L. M., S. L. Rauch, and R. K. Pitman. "Amygdala, Medial Prefrontal Cortex, and Hippocampal Function in PTSD," *Ann. NY Acad. Sci.* 1071 (July 2006), 67–79.

Shmist, Y. A., I. Goncharov, M. Eichler, V. Shneyvays, A. Isaac, Z. Vogel, and A. Shainberg. "Delta-9-Tetrahydrocannabinol Protects Cardiac Cells from Hypoxia via CB2 Receptor Activation and Nitric Oxide Production," *Mol. Cell Biochem.* 283:1–2 (February 2006), 75–83.

Shoval, G., L. Shbiro, L. Hershkovitz, N. Hazut, G. Zalsman, R. Mechoulam, and A. Weller. "Prohedonic Effect of Cannabidiol in a Rat Model of Depression," *Neuropsychobiology* 73:2 (2016),123–9.

Shurman, J., G. F. Koob, and H. B. Gutstein. "Opioids, Pain, the Brain, and Hyperkatifeia: A Framework for the Rational Use of Opioids for Pain," *Pain Medicine* 11:7 (2010), 1092–98.

Silva, P., and W. Stanton. *From Child to Adult: The Dunedin Multidisciplinary Health and Development Study*. Oxford, UK: Oxford University Press, 1996.

Simantov, R., and S. H. Snyder. "Morphine-like Peptides in Mammalian Brain: Isolation, Structure Elucidation, and Interactions with the Opiate Receptor," *Proceedings of the National Academy of Sciences of the United States of America* 73:7 (July 1976), 2515–19.

Sites, B. D., M. L. Beach, and M. Davis. "Increases in the Use of Prescription Opioid Analgesics and the Lack of Improvement in Disability Metrics Among Users," *Regional Anesthesia and Pain Medicine* 39:1 (2014), 6–12.

Slivicki, R. A., Z. Xu, P. M. Kulkarni, R. G. Pertwee, K. Mackie, G. A. Thakur, and A. G. Hohmann. "Positive Allosteric Modulation of Cannabinoid Receptor Type 1 Suppresses Pathological Pain Without Producing Tolerance or Dependence," *Biol. Psychiatry* pii: S0006-3223:17 (July 8, 2017), 31761–64.

Sloan, M. E., J. L. Gowin, V. A. Ramchandani, Y. L. Hurd, and B. Le Foll. "The Endocannabinoid System as a Target for Addiction Treatment: Trials and Tribulations," *Neuropharmacology* 124 (September 15, 2017), 73–83, Reiman et al., "Cannabis as a Substitute".

Small, E., and H. D. Beckstead. "Cannabinoid Phenotypes in *Cannabis sativa,*" *Nature* 245 (1973), 147–48.

———. "Common Cannabinoid Phenotypes in 350 Stocks of Cannabis," *Lloydia* 36 (1973), 144–65.

Smith, H. S., and P. D. Meek. "Pain Responsiveness to Opioids: Central Versus Peripheral Neuropathic Pain," *J. Opioid Manag.* 7:5 (September–October 2011), 391–400.

Smith, Philip H., Gregory G. Homish, R. Lorraine Collins, Gary A. Giovino, Helene R. White, and Kenneth E. Leonard. "Couples' Marijuana Use Is Inversely Related to Their Intimate Partner Violence over the First Nine Years of Marriage," *Psychol. Addict. Behav.* 28:3 (September 2014), 734–42.

Sommer, Claudia. "Peripheral Neuropathies: Long-Term Opioid Therapy in Neuropathy: Benefit or Harm?" *Nature Reviews Neurology* 13 (2017), 516–17.

Spampinato, U., E. Esposito, S. Romandini, et al. "Changes of Serotonin and Dopamine Metabolism in Various Forebrain Areas of Rats Injected with Morphine Either Systemically or in the Raphe Nuclei Dorsalis and Medianis," *Brain Res.* 328 (1985), 89–95.

Srivastava, M. D., B. I. Srivastava, and B. Brouhard. "D9-Tetrahydrocannabinol and Cannabidiol Alter Cytokine Production by Human Immune Cells, *Immunopharmacology* 40:3 (1998), 179–85.

Stanley, L. R., S. D. Harness, R. C. Swaim, F. Beauvais. "Rates of Substance Use of American Indian Students in 8th, 10th, and 12th Grades Living on or Near Reservations: Update, 2009–2012," *Public Health Reports* 129:2 (2014), 156–63.

Starowicz, K., W. Makuch, M. Osikowicz, F. Piscitelli, S. Petrosino, V. Di Marzo, and B. Przewlocka. "Spinal Anandamide Produces Analgesia in Neuropathic Rats: Possible CB(1)- and TRPV1-Mediated Mechanisms," *Neuropharmacology* 62:4 (March 2012), 1746–55.

Stein, C. "Targeting Pain and Inflammation by Peripherally Acting Opioids," *Frontiers in Pharmacology* 4 (2013), 123.

Stevens, A. J., and M. D. Higgins. "A Systematic Review of the Analgesic Efficacy of Cannabinoid Medications in the Management of Acute Pain," *Acta Anaesthesiol. Scand.* 61:3 (March 2017), 268–80.

Stevens, C. W., K. K. Martin, and B. W. Stahlheber. "Nociceptin Produces Antinociception after Spinal Administration in Amphibians," *Pharmacology, Biochemistry, and Behavior* 91:3 (2009), 436–40.

Storr, M. A., C. M. Keenan, D. Emmerdinger, H. Zhang, B. Yüce, A. Sibaev, F. Massa, et al. "Targeting Endocannabinoid Degradation Protects against Experimental Colitis in Mice: Involvement of CB(1) and CB(2) Receptors," *J. Mol. Med.* (Berl). 86:8 (August 2008), 925–36.

Strasser, F., D. Luftner, K. Possinger, G. Ernst, T. Ruhstaller, W. Meissner, Y. D. Ko, et al. "Comparison of Orally Administered Cannabis Extract and Delta-9 Tetrahydrocannabinol in Treating Patients with Cancer-Related Anorexia-Cachexia Syndrome: A Multicenter, Phase III, Randomized, Double-Blind, Placebo-Controlled Clinical Trial from the Cannabis-in-Cachexia-Study-Group," *J. Clin. Oncol.* 24:21 (2006), 3394–3400.

Strathdee, S. A., and C. Beyrer. "Threading the Needle—How to Stop the HIV Outbreak in Rural Indiana," *New England Journal of Medicine* 373:5 (2015), 397–9.

Streeter, C. C., J. E. Jensen, R. M. Perlmutter, H. J. Cabral, H. Tian, D. B. Terhune, D. A. Ciraulo, and P. F. Renshaw. "Yoga Asana Sessions Increase Brain GABA Levels: A Pilot Study," *J. Altern. Complement. Med.* 13:4 (May 2007), 419–26.

Strube, G. "Mittheilung über therapeutische Versuche mit Heroin," *Klinische Wochenschrift* 1898, 38.

Sumariwalla, P. F., R. Gallily, S. Tchilibon, E. Fride, R. Mechoulam, and M. Feldmann. "A Novel Synthetic, Nonpsychoactive Cannabinoid Acid (HU-320) with Antiinflammatory Properties in Murine Collagen-Induced Arthritis," *Arthritis Rheum.* 50:3 (2004), 985–998.

Swift, Wendy, Peter Gates, and Paul Dillon. "Survey of Australians Using Cannabis for Medical Purposes," *Harm Reduct. J.* 2 (2005), 18.

Sydenham, Thomas. *The Works of Thomas Sydenham,* trans. R. G. Latham (London: Sydenham Society, 1848), vol. I, xcix.

Szabo, B., U. Nordheim, and N. Niederhoffer. "Effects of Cannabinoids on Sympathetic and Parasympathetic Neuro-effector Transmission in the Rabbit Heart," *J. Pharmacol. Exp. Ther.* 297 (2001), 819–26.

Takahashi, R. N., and I. G. Karniol. "Pharmacologic Interaction between Cannabinol and Delta-9-Tetrahydrocannabinol," *Psychopharmacologia* 41:3 (1975), 277–84.

Takeda, S., N. Usami, I. Yamamoto, and K. Watanabe. "Cannabidiol-2',6'-Dimethyl Ether, a Cannabidiol Derivative, Is a Highly Potent and Selective 15 Lipoxygenase Inhibitor," *Drug Metab. Dispos.* 37:8 (August 2009), 1733–37.

Tambe, Y., H. Tsujiuchi, G. Honda, Y. Ikeshiro, and S. Tanaka. "Gastric Cytoprotection of the nonSteroidal Anti-inflammatory Sesquiterpene, Beta-Caryophyllene," *Planta Med.* 62:5 (October 1996), 469–70.

Tamura, Y., Y. Iwasaki, M. Narukawa, and T. Watanabe. "Ingestion of Cinnamaldehyde, a TRPA1 Agonist, Reduces Visceral Fats in Mice Fed a High-Fat and High-Sucrose Diet," *J. Nutr. Sci. Vitaminol.* (Tokyo) 58:1 (2012), 9–13.

Tart, Charles T. "Marijuana Intoxication: Common Experiences," *Nature* 226:5247 (May 1970), 701–4.

Tashkin, D. P., S. Reiss, B. J. Shapiro, B. Calvarese, J. L. Olsen, and J. W. Lodge. "Bronchial Effects of Aerosolized Delta 9-Tetrahydrocannabinol in Healthy and Asthmatic Subjects," *Am. Rev. Respir. Dis.* 115:1 (January 1977), 57–65.

Taylor, Bradley K., and Allan I. Basbaum. "Systemic Morphine-Induced Release of Serotonin in the Rostroventral Medulla is Not Mimicked by Morphine Microinjection into the Periaqueductal Gray," *Journal of Neurochemistry* 86 (2003), 1129–41.

Terry, C. E. *The Opium Problem.* New York: Bureau of Social Hygiene, 1928, 54.

Thompson, G. R., H. Rosenkrantz, U. H. Schaeppi, and M. C. Braude. "Comparison of Acute Oral Toxicity of Cannabinoids in Rats, Dogs and Monkeys," *Toxicol. Appl. Pharmacol.* 25 (1973), 363–72.

Tiihonen, J., M. Lehti, M. Aaltonen, et al. "Psychotropic Drugs and Homicide: A Prospective Cohort Study from Finland," *World Psychiatry* 14:2 (2015), 245–47.

Trancas, B., N. Borja Santos, and L. D. Patrício. "The Use of Opium in Roman Society and the Dependence of Princeps Marcus Aurelius," *Acta Med Port* 21:6 (November-December 2008), 581–90.

Trezza, Viviana, and Louk J. M. J. Vanderschuren. "Divergent Effects of Anandamide Transporter Inhibitors with Different Target Selectivity on Social Play Behavior in Adolescent Rats," *JPET* 328:1 (January 2009), 343–50.

Tringale, Rolando, and Claudia Jensen. "Cannabis and Insomnia," *O'Shaughnessy's* Autumn 2011, 31–32.

Tripathi, H. L., F. J. Vocci, D. A. Brase, and W. L. Dewey. "Effects of Cannabinoids on Levels of Acetylcholine and Choline and on Turnover Rate of Acetylcholine in Various Regions of the Mouse Brain," *Alcohol Drug Res.* 7:5–6 (1987), 525–32.

Tschirch, A. *Handbuch der Pharmakognosie I/III,* 1933, 1208, 1209.

Tsigos, C., and G. P. Chrousos. "Hypothalamic-Pituitary-Adrenal Axis, Neuroendocrine Factors and Stress," *J. Psychosom. Res.* 53:4 (October 2002), 865–71.

Tutu, Desmond. "Apartheid, Perpetrators, Forgiveness: Desmond Tutu's Views," www.youtube .com/watch?v=eRDBWoV_hA0.

U.S. Centers for Disease Control and Prevention (CDC). "Alcohol-Attributable Deaths and Years of Potential Life Lost—United States, 2001," *MMWR* 53:37 (September 24, 2004), 866–70.

———. "Provisional Counts of Overdose Deaths, as of August 6, 2017," www.cdc.gov/nchs /data/health_policy/monthly-drug-overdose-death-estimates.pdf.

———. "Smoking-Attributable Mortality, Years of Potential Life Lost, and Productivity Losses—United States, 2000–2004," *MMWR* 57:45 (November 14, 2008), 1226–28.

———. "Today's Heroin Epidemic Infographics," Vital Signs, www.cdc.gov/vitalsigns/heroin /infographic.html.

U.S. Department of Health and Human Services, Substance Abuse and Mental Health Services Administration. *Mortality Data from the Drug Abuse Warning Network, 2002.* Rockville, MD: NCADI, 2002.

U.S. Department of Justice, Office of Public Affairs. "AlphaBay, the Largest Online 'Dark Market,' Shut Down," July 20, 2017, www.justice.gov/opa/pr/alphabay-largest-online -dark-market-shut-down.

U.S. Drug Enforcement Agency (DEA). *Headquarters News,* September 22, 2016, www.dea.gov /divisions/hq/2016/hq092216.shtml.

U.S. Drug Enforcement Agency, Miami Division. "Miami News: Florida Doctors No Longer Among the Top Oxycodone Purchasers in the United States," April 5, 2013, www.dea.gov /divisions/mia/2013/mia040513.shtml.

U.S. Food and Drug Administration, Office of the Commissioner. "Press Announcements: FDA Requests Removal of Opana ER for Risks Related to Abuse," www.fda.gov. Accessed June 15, 2017.

Ulugol, A., H. C. Karadag, Y. Ipci, M. Tamer, and I. Dokmeci. "The Effect of WIN 55,212- 2, a Cannabinoid Agonist, on Tactile Allodynia in Diabetic Rats," *Neurosci. Lett.* 371:2–3 (November 23, 2004), 167–70.

Usami, Noriyuki, Takeshi Okuda, Hisatoshi Yoshida, Toshiyuki Kimura, Kazuhito Watanabe, Hidetoshi Yoshimura, and Ikuo Yamamoto. "Synthesis and Pharmacological Evaluation in Mice of Halogenated Cannabidiol Derivatives," *Chem. Pharm. Bull.* 47:11 (1999), 1641–45.

Utomo, W. K., M. de Vries, H. Braat, et al. "Modulation of Human Peripheral Blood Mononuclear Cell Signaling by Medicinal Cannabinoids," *Frontiers in Molecular Neuroscience* 10 (2017), 14.

Valverde, O., F. Noble, F. Beslot, V. Daugé, M. C. Fournié-Zaluski, and B. P. Roques. "Delta9-Tetrahydrocannabinol Releases and Facilitates the Effects of Endogenous Enkephalins: Reduction in Morphine Withdrawal Syndrome without Change in Rewarding Effect," *Eur. J. Neurosci.* 13:9 (May 2001), 1816–24.

Van Dam, D., E. Vedel, T. Ehring, and P. M. G. Emmelkamp. "Psychological Treatments for Concurrent Posttraumatic Stress Disorder and Substance Use Disorder: A Systematic Review," *Clinical Psychology Review* 32 (2012), 202–14.

Vela, G., M. Ruiz-Gayo, and J. A. Fuentes. "Anandamide Decreases Naloxone-Precipitated Withdrawal Signs in Mice Chronically Treated with Morphine," *Neuropharmacology* 34:6 (June 1995), 665–68.

Vin-Raviv, N., T. Akinyemiju, Q. Meng, S. Sakhuja, and R. Hayward. "Marijuana Use and Inpatient Outcomes among Hospitalized Patients: Analysis of the Nationwide Inpatient Sample Database," *Cancer Med.* 6:1 (January 2017), 320–29.

Vitalo, A., J. Fricchione, M. Casali, Y. Berdichevsky, E. A. Hoge, S. L. Rauch, F. Berthiaume, et al. "Nest-Making and Oxytocin Comparably Promote Wound Healing in Isolation-Reared Rats." *PLoS One* 4:5 (2009), e5523.

Volpi-Abadie, J., A. M. Kaye, and A. D. Kaye. "Serotonin Syndrome," *The Ochsner Journal* 13:4 (2013), 533–40.

von Hippel, William, Loren Brener, and Courtney von Hippel. "Implicit Prejudice Toward Injecting Drug Users Predicts Intentions to Change Jobs Among Drug and Alcohol Nurses," *Psychological Science* 19:1 (January 2008), 7–11.

Vowles, K. E., M. L. McEntee, P. S. Julnes, T. Frohe, J. P. Ney, and D. N. van der Goes. "Rates of Opioid Misuse, Abuse, and Addiction in Chronic Pain: A Systematic Review and Data Synthesis," *Pain* 156:4 (April 2015), 569–76.

Wade, D. T., P. Robson, H. House, et al. "A Preliminary Controlled Study to Determine Whether Whole-Plant Cannabis Extracts Can Improve Intractable Neurogenic Symptoms," *Clin. Rehabil.* 17:1 (2003), 18–26.

Waldman, M., E. Hochhauser, M. Fishbein, D. Aravot, A. Shainberg, and Y. Sarne. "An Ultralow Dose of Tetrahydrocannabinol Provides Cardioprotection," *Biochem. Pharmacol.* 85:11 (June 1, 2013), 1626–33.

Walker, J. M., and A. G. Hohmann. "Cannabinoid Mechanisms of Pain Suppression," Handb. Exp. Pharmacol. 168 (2005), 509–54.

Walker, Winifred. *The Plants of the Bible*. London: Lutterworth, 1959.

Wallace, M. S., T. D. Marcotte, A. Umlauf, B. Gouaux, and J. H. Atkinson. "Efficacy of Inhaled Cannabis on Painful Diabetic Neuropathy," *J. Pain* 16:7 (July 2015), 616–27.

Walsh, S. K., C. Y. Hepburn, K. A. Kane, and C. L. Wainwright. "Acute Administration of Cannabidiol In Vivo Suppresses Ischaemia-Induced Cardiac Arrhythmias and Reduces Infarct Size When Given at Reperfusion," *British Journal of Pharmacology* 160:5 (2010), 1234–42.

Walter, M., D. Bentz N. Schicktanz, A. Milnik, A. Aerni, C. Gerhards, K. Schwegler, et al. "Effects of Cortisol Administration on Craving in Heroin Addicts," *Translational Psychiatry* 5 (2015), e610.

Walther, S., R. Mahlberg, U. Eichmann, and D. Kunz. "Delta-9-Tetrahydrocannabinol for Nighttime Agitation in Severe Dementia," *Psychopharmacology* (Berl). 185:4 (May 2006), 524–28.

Wand, G. "The Influence of Stress on the Transition From Drug Use to Addiction," *Alcohol Research & Health* 31:2 (2008), 119–36.

Ware, M. A., T. Wang, S. Shapiro, and J. P. Collet. "Cannabis for the Management of Pain: Assessment of Safety Study (COMPASS)," *Journal of Pain* 16:12 (2015), 1233–42.

Washington Post, "The FDA Takes a Stand Against an Opioid that Fueled an Epidemic," *The Washington Post*, June 12, 2017.

Watterson, G., R. Howard, and A. Goldman. "Peripheral Opioids in Inflammatory Pain," *Archives of Disease in Childhood* 89:7 (2004), 679–81.

Wei, Don, DaYeon Lee, Conor D. Cox, Carley A. Karsten, Olga Peñagarikano, Daniel H. Geschwind, Christine M. Gall, and Daniele Piomellia. "Endocannabinoid Signaling Mediates Oxytocin-Driven Social Reward," *PNAS* 112:45 (October 26, 2015), 14084–89.

Weiss, L., M. Zeira, S. Reich, S. Slavin, I. Raz, R. Mechoulam, and R. Gallily. "Cannabidiol arrests onset of autoimmune diabetes in NOD mice," *Neuropharmacology* 54: 1 (January 2008), 244–49.

Werb, Dan, Thomas Kerr, Bohdan Nosyk, Steffanie Strathdee, Julio Montaner, and Evan Wood. "The Temporal Relationship between Drug Supply Indicators: An Audit of International Government Surveillance Systems," *BMJ Open* 3:9 (September 30, 2013).

Wilkerson, Jenny L., and Erin D. Milligan. "The Central Role of Glia in Pathological Pain and the Potential of Targeting the Cannabinoid 2 Receptor for Pain Relief," *ISRN Anesthesiology* 2011 (2011), article ID 593894.

Williams, E., B. Stewart-Knox, A. Helander, C. McConville, I. Bradbury, and I. Rowland. "Associations Between Whole-Blood Serotonin and Subjective Mood in Healthy Male Volunteers," *Biol. Psychol.* 71:2 (February 2006), 171–74.

Williams, S. J., J. P. Hartley, and J. D. Graham. "Bronchodilator Effect of Delta1-Tetrahydrocannabinol Administered by Aerosol of Asthmatic Patients," *Thorax* 31:6 (1976), 720–23.

Willoughby, Karen A., Sandra F. Moore, Billy R. Martin, and Earl F. Ellis. "The Biodisposition and Metabolism of Anandamide in Mice," *Journal of Pharmacology and Experimental Therapeutics* 282:1 (July 1997), 243–47.

Wilsey, B., T. D. Marcotte, R. Deutsch, H. Zhao, H. Prasad, and A. Phan. "An Exploratory Human Laboratory Experiment Evaluating Vaporized Cannabis in the Treatment of Neuropathic Pain from Spinal Cord Injury and Disease," *Journal of Pain* 17:9 (2016), 982–1000.

Wilsey, B., T. Marcotte, A. Tsodikov, J. Millman, H. Bentley, B. Gouaux, and S. Fishman. "A Randomized, Placebo-Controlled, Crossover Trial of Cannabis Cigarettes in Neuropathic Pain," *J. Pain* 9:6 (June 2008), 506–21.

Wilsey, Barth, Thomas D. Marcotte, Reena Deutsch, Ben Gouaux, Staci Sakai, and Haylee Donaghe. "Low Dose Vaporized Cannabis Significantly Improves Neuropathic Pain," *J. Pain* 14:2 (February 2013), 136–48.

Wilson, M. M., C. Philpot, and J. E. Morley. "Anorexia of Aging in Long-Term Care: Is Dronabinol an Effective Appetite Stimulant?—a Pilot Study," *J. Nutr. Health Aging* 11:2 (March–April 2007), 195–98.

Wilson, N. M., H. Jung, M. S. Ripsch, R. J. Miller, and F. A. White. "CXCR4 Signaling Mediates Morphine-Induced Tactile Hyperalgesia," *Brain Behav. Immun.* 25 (2011), 565–73.

Winchester, W. J., K. Gore, S. Glatt, W. Petit, J. C. Gardiner, K. Conlon, M. Postlethwaite, et al. "Inhibition of TRPM8 Channels Reduces Pain in the Cold Pressor Test in Humans," *Pharmacol. Exp. Ther.* 351:2 (November 2014), 259–69.

Wisniak, Jaime. "Pierre-Jean Robiquet," *Educación Química* 24 (S1: March 2013), 139–49.

Witvliet, C. V., T. E. Ludwig, and D. J. Bauer. "Please Forgive Me: Transgressors' Emotions and Physiology during Imagery of Seeking Forgiveness and Victim Responses," *Journal of Psychology and Christianity* 21 (2002), 219–33.

Wohl, Anthony S. *Endangered Lives: Public Health in Victorian Britain.* Cambridge, MA: Harvard University Press, 1983.

Woolf, C. J. "What Is This Thing Called Pain?" *Journal of Clinical Investigation* 120:11 (2010), 3742–44.

World Health Organization. "WHO's Pain Ladder," 2011, www.who.int/cancer/palliative/painladder/en.

Wright, C. R. A. "On the Action of Organic Acids and their Anhydrides on the Natural Alkaloids," *Journal of the Chemical Society* 27 (1874), 1031–43.

Wright, S., P. Duncombe, D. G. Altman. "Assessment of Blinding to Treatment Allocation in Studies of a Cannabis-Based Medicine (Sativex) in People with Multiple Sclerosis: A New Approach," *Trials* 13 (2012), 189.

Xu, Nan-Jie, Lan Bao, Hua-Ping Fan, Guo-Bin Bao, Lu Pu, Ying-Jin Lu, Chun-Fu Wu, et al. "Morphine Withdrawal Increases Glutamate Uptake and Surface Expression of Glutamate Transporter GLT1 at Hippocampal Synapses," *Journal of Neuroscience* 23:11 (June 1, 2003), 4775–84.

Yamaguchi, T., Y. Hagiwara, H. Tanaka, T. Sugiura, K. Waku, Y. Shoyama, S. Watanabe, and T. Yamamoto. "Endogenous Cannabinoid, 2-Arachidonoylglycerol, Attenuates Naloxone-Precipitated Withdrawal Signs in Morphine-Dependent Mice," *Brain Res.* 909:1–2 (August 3, 2001), 121–26.

Yang, J., Y. Yang, J. M. Chen, W. Y. Liu, C. H. Wang, and B. C. Lin. "Central Oxytocin Enhances Antinociception in the Rat," *Peptides* 28:5 (May 2007), 1113–19.

Yi, H., T. Iida, S. Liu, D. Ikegami, Q. Liu, A. Iida, D. A. Lubarsky, and S. Hao. "IL-4 Mediated by HSV Vector Suppresses Morphine Withdrawal Response and Decreases TNFα, NR2B, and pC/EBPβ in the Periaqueductal Gray in Rats," *Gene Therapy* 24 (April 2017), 224–33.

Zak, P. J., A. A. Stanton, and S. Ahmadi. "Oxytocin Increases Generosity in Humans," *PLoS One* 2:11 (November 7, 2007), e1128.

Zhang, Z., C. Yang, X. Dai, Y. Ao, and Y. Li. "Inhibitory Effect of Trans-Caryophyllene (TC) on Leukocyte-Endothelial Attachment," *Toxicol. Appl. Pharmacol.* 329 (June 15, 2017), 326–33.

Zhao, Y., Z. Yuan, Y. Liu, J. Xue, Y. Tian, W. Liu, W. Zhang, et. al. "Activation of Cannabinoid CB2 Receptor Ameliorates Atherosclerosis Associated with Suppression of Adhesion Molecules," *J. Cardiovasc. Pharmacol.* 9 (January 2010).

Zheng, Yangwen. "The Art of Alchemists, Sex, and Court Ladies," in *The Social Life of Opium in China.* Cambridge, UK: Cambridge University Press, 2005.

Ziegler, C. G., C. Mohn, V. Lamounier-Zepter, V. Rettori, S. R. Bornstein, A. W. Krug, and M. Ehrhart-Bornstein. "Expression and Function of Endocannabinoid Receptors in the Human Adrenal Cortex," *Horm. Metab. Res.* 42:2 (Februar 2010), 88–92.

Ziring, D., B. Wei, P. Velazquez, M. Schrage, N. E. Buckley, and J. Braun. "Formation of B and T Cell Subsets Require the Cannabinoid Receptor CB2," *Immunogenetics.* 58 (2006), 714–25.

Zuardi, A., J. Crippa, S. Dursun, S. Morais, J. Vilela, R. Sanches, and J. Hal-lak. "Cannabidiol Was Ineffective for Manic Episode of Bipolar Affective Disorder," *J. Psychopharmacol.* 24:1 (January 2010), 135–37.

Zubieta, J. K., Y. R. Smith, J. A. Bueller, Y. Xu, M. R. Kilbourn, D. M. Jewett, C. R. Meyer, R. A. Koeppe, and C. S. Stohler, "Regional Mu Opioid Receptor Regulation of Sensory and Affective Dimensions of Pain," *Science* 293 (2001), 311–15.

ACKNOWLEDGMENTS

I want to thank everyone at North Atlantic Books who contributed to the realization of this book. Following my first book, *Cannabis Health Index,* my initial concept and idea for what I wanted to write about next was too broad, and in its early stages lacked precision and focus. However, publisher Tim McKee provided feedback from the acquisitions group that ultimately excited and encouraged me to sharpen the timely message of the current book. Thanks to acquisition editor Vanessa Ta who got the practical ball rolling; to editor Kathy Glass for her editing skills informed by an abundance of cannabis-culture wisdom; to project editor Louis Swaim for paying attention to details, for his effective diplomatic skills in navigating the graphics, endnotes, and index, and for seeing the project through its delivery; and finally to copyeditor Christopher Church for going over the manuscript with a fine-toothed comb, assuring good form and readability.

INDEX

ABOUT THE AUTHOR

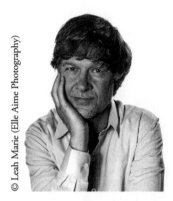

UWE BLESCHING is a medical writer and regular contributor to the cannabinoid health sciences, mind-body medicine, phytopharmacology, as well as evidence-based illness prevention and treatment protocols. In addition to his life-long passion for integrative medicine, his latest book *Breaking the Cycle of Opioid Addiction: Supplement Your Pain Management with Cannabis* is informed by rigorous in-depth research and twenty years' experience in emergency medicine as a paramedic for the City of San Francisco. He holds a BA in humanities from the New College of California, an MA in psychology, and a PhD in higher education and social change from the Western Institute for Social Research.

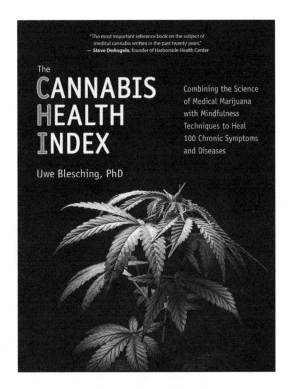

The Cannabis Health Index
978-1-58394-962-7

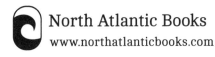

North Atlantic Books
www.northatlanticbooks.com

North Atlantic Books is an independent, nonprofit publisher committed to a bold exploration of the relationships between mind, body, spirit, and nature.

About North Atlantic Books

North Atlantic Books (NAB) is an independent, nonprofit publisher committed to a bold exploration of the relationships between mind, body, spirit, and nature. Founded in 1974, NAB aims to nurture a holistic view of the arts, sciences, humanities, and healing. To make a donation or to learn more about our books, authors, events, and newsletter, please visit www.northatlanticbooks.com.

North Atlantic Books is the publishing arm of the Society for the Study of Native Arts and Sciences, a 501(c)(3) nonprofit educational organization that promotes cross-cultural perspectives linking scientific, social, and artistic fields. To learn how you can support us, please visit our website.